LYMPHOEDEMA

Methods of Treatment and Control

A GUIDE FOR PATIENTS
AND THERAPISTS

By
Prof. Michael Földi MD
and
Ethel Földi MD

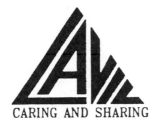

CARING AND SHARING

Translated from the original German – 'Das Lymphödem' – 5th Edition

By

Dr. Andrew C. Newell MA MD FRACP

for the

LYMPHOEDEMA ASSOCIATION of VICTORIA Inc – AUSTRALIA

Reproduced with the kind permission of the Authors and with the approval
of the Publishers – Gustav Fischer Verlag – Stuttgart – New York

Földi/Földi, "Das Lymphödem", 5th Edition
GUSTAV FISCHER VERLAG – Stuttgart – (c) 1991

Published by: Lymphoedema Association of Victoria
                 50 St. Georges Rd.
                 Upper Beaconsfield, Victoria 3808
                 Australia

Printed by: modcoprint
                 8 Manton Road
                 Oakleigh South, Victoria 3167
                 Australia

Lymphoedema Association of Victoria
ISBN 0 646 22342 9

Reprinted with the kind permission of the Lymphoedema Association of Victoria by:

MEDICINA BIOLOGICA
2937 NE Flanders St.
Portland, OR 97232
Tel: (503) 287-6775
Fax: (503) 235-3520

THE AUTHORS

Professor Michael Földi graduated in medicine in Hungary and worked as Professor of Internal Medicine in the University of Szeged, where he concentrated on intensive research in basic lymphology. His findings have been published in numerous scientific articles, monographs and books.

After he escaped from Hungary in 1969 he spent most of his professional life working in the Federal Republic of Germany investigating, treating and teaching in the field of lymphology.

Professor Földi works with his wife, Dr. Ethel Földi in the Földi Clinic in the picturesque Black Forest town of Hinterzarten, in the vicinity of Freiburg/Breisgau. In this idyllic setting he has applied his principles of combined physical therapy to management of those suffering from lymphoedema, in particular women who have undergone surgery or radiotherapy for carcinoma of the breast along with many other types of lymphoedema occurring in the course of cancer treatment in women and men, and lymphoedemas of different origin.

In addition, Professor Földi directs the activities of the Földi schools in Berlin, Freiburg and Munich where approximately 8,000 therapists have been trained to carry out the specialised techniques required to manage lymphoedema.

Continues next page

THE TRANSLATOR

Dr. Andrew Colgate Newell graduated from the University of Melbourne with the degrees of Bachelor of Medicine and Bachelor of Surgery in 1944 and Doctor of Medicine in 1949. He was elected to Fellowship of the Royal Australasian College of Physicians in 1963 and continues to practice as a consultant physician.

Because of his interest in European languages he returned to the University of Melbourne to complete B.A. (Hons) in 1983 and M.A. in 1989 in the School of Germanic Studies. His M.A. thesis was based on a study of translations into Old Norse of the 12th century 'romans courtois'.

ACKNOWLEDGEMENTS

A generous loan to cover the cost of the initial printing of the English translation of 'Das Lymphödem' was provided to the Lymphoedema Association of Victoria Inc. by Beiersdorf Australia Pty. Ltd. via the Lymphoedema Practitioner's Education Group of Victoria.

An additional repayable loan to enable the purchase of the photographic duplicates of the illustrations contained in the German edition of 'Das Lymphödem' was granted to the Lymphoedema Association of Victoria Inc. by the Lymphoedema Association of Australia Inc.

THE LYMPHOEDEMA ASSOCIATION of VICTORIA Inc.
AND THE ENGLISH TRANSLATION OF
"DAS LYMPHÖDEM – LYMPHOEDEMA"

The Lymphoedema Association of Victoria Incorporated (L.A. of Vic.) was formed in June 1990. Two of its main aims are to collect and distribute information on lymphoedema and to provide personal support and encouragement to those who have the condition.

One of the founding members of the L.A. of Vic. underwent treatment at the Földiklinik in Hinterzarten, Germany. Before returning to Australia after completing her course of treatment, she purchased a copy of the German edition of "Das Lymphödem". The Committee saw an obvious need for an English translation of this valuable text which could, hopefully, be made available in all English-speaking countries. Dr. Andrew Newell was suggested as the most appropriate person to perform the translation, and he graciously consented to undertake the task on behalf of the L.A. of Vic.

Our sincere thanks are extended to Dr. Newell for his very considerable voluntary efforts on behalf of the L.A. of Vic., and to Professor and Frau Földi for their agreement and encouragement to proceed with the project. Gustav Fischer Verlag have kindly given the Association permission to publish the English translation, and we are most appreciative of their support and assistance during the negotiation of the terms of that contract.

Julia Wurf   March 1993

FOREWORD TO THE FIRST EDITION

Lymphology is the step-child of medicine. The universities offer doctors in training neither the requisite knowledge of anatomy and physiology nor their clinical application. Lymphology is sadly neglected in post-graduate education. The burden is carried by the patient who has lymphoedema and who very often remains without care. The doctor, endowed with scant knowledge, comforts his patient that he or she will have to come to terms with their condition. Unfortunately it can also happen that, in spite of scientific ignorance, investigations are carried out which lead to no therapeutic gain but may even do harm, and major operations are performed which in the overwhelming majority of cases are avoidable and, not uncommonly, are harmful. In our clinic we are asked every day by our patients "Why was I not informed by my doctor ?" "Why was I not referred in the first place for such effective conservative treatment; why did I have to find out about your clinic from my neighbor (or Radio Luxembourg)?". The lymphoedema sufferer hungers for information, and the need for counselling is, in this respect, far more pressing than for those who represent the "spoilt children" of medicine - as for example high blood pressure, arteriosclerosis or cancer.

In this respect lymphology has an extraordinarily close correlation with oncology. Most cases of lymphoedema arise following surgery or radiotherapy for a malignant tumour, but in addition many cases are directly caused by malignancy. On the other hand, neglected lymphoedema in the stage of so-called elephantiasis runs the risk of sarcomatous degeneration. In spite of this it is true, unfortunately, that the oncologist scarcely concerns himself with the lymphological aspects of after-care and surveillance of cancer. Scientific congresses devoted to oncology tend to ignore lymphology.

We ask our readers to consider this book as a structural entity. For example, if those who suffer from lymphoedema of the leg seek to be informed about their problem, it is not sufficient merely to limit their reading to one small chapter; they should start at the beginning. Without knowledge of the normal functioning of the lymphatic system, without a general awareness of the consequences of lymph stasis, they will not understand their particular illness. Because of the comparative frequency of lymphoedema of the arm following surgery or radiotherapy for breast cancer, we have developed this chapter in greater detail. Nevertheless, when writing this chapter we have all our readers in mind.

We hope that this little book will serve the lymphoedema sufferers, and also that interested doctors will gain something from its reading.

Michael Földi and Ethel Földi.

FOREWORD TO THE FIFTH EDITION

After only fifteen months, the fourth edition of this manual for patients is out of print. We believe that we can conclude from this fact that the work will be read not only by patients, but by doctors as well as the masseurs, physiotherapists, hydrotherapists and remedial gymnasts involved in Combined Physical Therapy for the reduction of oedema.

The fifth edition which now follows has been further improved and updated. This has involved not only the text, but also the list of therapists now classified by postal district. Since January 1989, when we completed the manuscript of the fourth edition, the number of graduates who have passed out of our two training schools in Freiburg and Munich has been increased by about 1200. The reader can now refer to a list of therapists which, including former students, now totals 7200.

We have also brought up to date the list of Branch Presidents of the "Self help for women with cancer" groups in Germany.

We trust that this revised work will help our patients to understand their disease and its treatment, and prepare them for their every-day problems.

Hinderzarten/Freiburg, December 1990

Ethel and Michael Földi

PREFACE

The aim of any manual for use by patients is to promote understanding and the ability to face life courageously. If the work is written with the sensitivity and the persuasiveness of a practising doctor, it achieves this aim on the basis of that mutual trust and respect which enable doctor and patient together to overcome human suffering. In mastering any illness, what is of usual relevance gains a particular dimension in the case of malignant disease. This book highlights the fact that, without the conscious and active participation of the patient, optimal success in both therapy and rehabilitation cannot be achieved.

The success of this book, therefore, is that it fulfills in an exemplary manner the difficult and even more important task of providing information and, at the same time, intelligible direction for the non-medical reader without in any way departing from its value as a scientific text which alone would guarantee its acceptance as a serious medical guide. It presents far more than just an inventory of current medical knowledge. Directed towards those who have undergone surgery or radiotherapy, this book provides a precise guide for both the affected patient and the attending doctor. It allows patient and physician to cope with the pain and distress which characterizes the treatment and rehabilitation of malignant disease. The fact that the author casts a critical eye on present day treatment methods for cancer patients provides for the treating doctor a valuable addition to his existing armamentarium.

It is this frankness in particular which justifies the claim of this publication to be a guide, companion and help for cancer sufferers. I trust therefore that this book will evoke a response which, because of its intention to improve still futher the existing cooperation between doctor and patient, it richly deserves.

February 1983   Mildred Scheel

TABLE OF CONTENTS

continues page 16

APPENDICES

1. LYMPH AND THE LYMPHATICS IN HEALTH

Seventy times a minute "that special sap" (Goethe), the blood, is driven by the left ventricle of the heart into the aorta. From there it passes into a branching system of tubes which meander throughout the body. Of these, the smallest units of the blood circulation are represented by minute hair-like vessels - the capillaries - seen only under the microscope. In most organs these form an intricate network embedded in the connective tissue which lies between the cells - the so called interstitial layer. The circulating blood permits the passage of essential nutrients and oxygen, dissolved in water, through the capillary wall to supply the needs of the tissues and at the same time allows waste products and carbon dioxide to pass back into the circulation. Finally the blood flows by way of the veins to the right atrium of the heart, and thence into the right ventricle. From here it is pumped via the pulmonary arteries to the lungs.

In the pulmonary circulation too, there is branching and rebranching until a capillary network is formed. Carbon dioxide is given up and the blood replenished with oxygen. Oxygenated blood then flows through pulmonary veins to the left atrium and finally the left ventricle, and so the circulation is complete. In the arteries of the body the bright red oxygen rich blood (arterial blood) moves in a pulsatile manner, and in this way a tangible pulse is produced. Dark, poorly oxygenated "venous blood" flows quietly through the veins so that those lying superficially appear blue through the skin.

There is, however, an additional system of vessels in our body, namely the lymphatics, which acts like a drainage reticulation alongside arteries and veins. These lymph capillaries, or lymphatics, are also found in the interstitial layer. In contradistinction to blood vessels, the lymphatics are neither visible nor palpable except in certain disease states. In the presence of inflammation (lymphangitis), the lymphatic vessels are recognizable as one or more red streaks. The lymph which flows through these vessels is crystal clear. The exception is found only in the intestinal lymphatics. These are seen during an abdominal operation when a fatty meal has been eaten a short time earlier, because fat is transported

17

from the gut by way of lymphatics. Fat colours the lymph yellowish white ("chyle"), and this colour is readily seen through the thin walled lymphatics. Superficial lymphatics can be visualised by the injection of a blue pigment (patent blue dye) into an appropriate area of subcutaneous tissue. This pigment moves from the interstitial tissue into the lymphatics and colors the lymph. The capillary wall is so thin that its content can now readily be seen, glistening blue through the skin. In medical practice we use this procedure for diagnostic purposes, and by this simple process we can ascertain the quality and the functional state of the lymphatics. We will deal with this point later when discussing lymphoedema. If lymphography, so called, is required, our object can be achieved by making a small incision under local anaesthetic to expose the lymphatics rendered visible by this technique. A radiographic contrast medium is then injected into the lymphatic. In this way lymphatics and lymph nodes can be displayed.

In contrast to the blood circulation, which together with the heart forms an integrated closed system, the lymphatic system is merely half a system - the outflow part. Lymph capillaries lie in intimate relation to blood capillaries in much the same way as tree roots interlace. Collected from its various tributaries, the lymphatic system empties itself by way of two main trunks - the thoracic duct and the right lymphatic trunk - into the venous limb of the lesser circulation. This area, referred to as the *angulus venosus*, is located behind the left clavicle or collarbone and is formed by the junction of the left clavicular vein and the left internal jugular vein.

Blood flow is maintained by the pumping action of the heart but, on the other hand, lymph flow is brought about by the intrinsic activity of the lymphatics. Having reached a certain dimension, the walls of the lymphatics contain smooth muscle cells and nerves as well as valves, so directed that they allow exclusively a centripetal[1] flow of lymph.

According to the well known Swiss biologist *Mislin,* the segment of a lymphatic bounded by two sets of valves is termed a *lymphangion.*

(1) centripetal - in a central direction

18

Whenever lymph reaches a distal$_{(2)}$ segment, it excites a stretch reflex; the lymphangion contracts and the muscle mass squeezes the lymph contained in it to the nearest proximal$_{(3)}$ lymphangion. The individual *lymphangia* can be regarded as miniature lymph hearts. (There are animal species, like the frog, which have true self-initiating and rhythmically contracting "lymph hearts". Stasis within these lymph hearts permits the frog to interrupt lymph flow suddenly; the animal swells up like a balloon and sinks to the bottom.)

The function of the lymphangion is adapted to demands in a quite remarkable manner. In states of complete physical rest, only minimal lymph flow occurs in the limbs. If for any reason the lymphatic workload$_{(4)}$ increases, the minute volume of lymph flow also increases. By so doing, any increase in demand brings about a corresponding increase in frequency and amplitude of pulsation of the lymphangion. The pacemaker, that is the electrical impulse contained within the lymphatic wall, serves this purpose in much the same way as in our "big" heart.

There are several additional mechanisms which assist and maintain lymph flow. Whenever we move, our contracting muscles compress the lymphatics and drive the flow of lymph in the direction of the heart. Pulsating arteries in the vicinity of the lymphatics, as well as respiratory movement, play an accessory role in this "lymphokinetics"$_{(5)}$. An interesting characteristic of the lymphatics from capillary to thoracic duct consists of a significant degree of permeability of the lymphatic wall which, by removing water, progressively concentrates the lymph as it flows in a proximal direction - particularly when the pressure within the vessel is high. One other notable characteristic of the lymphatic system is the

---

(2)   *distal - from body or limbs*

(3)   *proximal: the direction of the trunk*

(4)   *lymphatic workload: the amount of protein and fluid which must be carried away from the tissue fluid by way of the lymphatic system*

(5)   *the Greek word kinein means to move; lymphokinetics = movement or flow of lymph.*

presence of lymph nodes which are interposed strategically between regions of the body.

Lymph nodes which are in relation to a part of the body or to an
organ are termed *"regional lymph nodes"*. These can be compared
to a purification plant; their task is to purify the lymph which
passes through them. In addition the lymph nodes share with
thymus, tonsils and spleen the function of production of the so-
called lymphocytes, cells which are extremely important in the
fight against infection and in the development of immunity. Table 1
shows that lymphocytes are already present in lymph flowing in the
so-called *afferent*(6) lymphatics. This means that a proportion of the
lymphocytes leave the capillary network of the blood and, passing
through the interstitial tissues, reach pores in the lymphatic wall.

TABLE 1. Migration of lymphocytes between spleen, lymph nodes, blood and lymph
nodes.

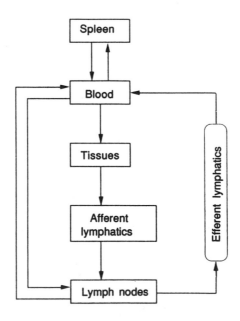

(6) *afferent: leading up to*

A percentage of lymphocytes traversing the nodes remain there, so that damaged or effete cells are destroyed. Another fraction passes through the node and exits by way of the *efferent*[7] lymphatics. However lymph in efferent lymphatics contains more lymphocytes than in the afferent lymphatics because, in their passage through the lymph node, two additional types of lymphocytes are added to it:

1) Lymphocytes which reach the lymph node through its intrinsic micro-circulation.

2) Lymphocytes arising solely in the nodes.

The ability of the nodes to store lymphocytes is one of their most interesting and unusual attributes. Lymph and lymphocytes can also be discharged directly into the blood circulation by way of the venules[8] which drain the nodes.

What then is the nature of this lymph?[9] Lymph arises from interstitial fluid (tissue fluid) but is in no way identical with it; this is still accepted in scientific circles.

As we know already, interstitial fluid arises from the blood. Together with blood, interstitial fluid and lymph also form part of the *"extra-cellular fluid compartment"* (Table 2).

TABLE 2. Fluid Compartments in the body

1.	Intracellular	2.2.1	Interstitial
2.	Extracellular	2.2.2	Cerebrospinal fluid
2.1	Intravascular	2.2.3	Endolymph and perilymph
2.1.1	Blood Interstitial	2.2.4	Chambers of the eye
2.1.2	Lymph	2.2.5	Joint cavities
2.2	Extravascular	2.2.6	Serous cavities of the body

In the production of interstitial fluid, as well as its maintenance in

(7) *efferent: leading away*

(8) *venule: a small vein*

(9) *the greco-latin work "lymph" means fluid as clear as water.*

and dispersal from the tissues, two processes play a part, namely *diffusion* and *filtration/absorption*. When one carefully overlayers a concentrated salt solution (e.g. common salt) with a less concentrated solution, salt molecules[10] migrate from the concentrated and into the less concentrated solution; the solvent (water) migrates in the opposite direction from the less concentrated to the more concentrated medium. This process is termed *diffusion.* If a membrane which has the ability to permit the passage of water but not salt is interposed between the more concentrated and the less concentrated solutions, naturally only water will pass through the barrier and enter the concentrated solution. Such a membrane is said to be semi-permeable. Due to the passage of water, a so-called osmotic[11] pressure arises in the chamber containing the more concentrated solution. Osmotic pressure represents the energy by which salt attracts water. If pressure is now exerted from the outside against the space containing the concentrated solution, one can overcome osmotic pressure; that is one can reverse the flow of water - we speak of *filtration.*

If we add a *protein solution* instead of a salt solution to a beaker and separate these by a membrane which allows free passage of water and salt but is impermeable to protein molecules (protein molecules are considerably larger than salt and water molecules) from a less concentrated solution, water can now move into the more concentrated protein solution and bring about the so-called *colloid*[12] *osmotic pressure.* Using this technique it is also possible to exert pressure on the concentrated protein solution and drive water back from the chamber with the high protein concentration into the one with the low protein concentration; we call this *ultrafiltration.* If one lowers the pressure to which the filtered fluid is exposed, the term is *vacuum ultrafiltration.*

The capillary wall corresponds to a membrane which is completely

(10) molecule: the smallest unit of chemical matter.

(11) osmotic: Greek osmos thrust, drive.

(12) Greek: kollo - clay

permeable to salt and water. There is no barrier to diffusion out of the circulation into the interstitial fluid and back again. However for blood proteins the capillary wall is largely impermeable.

FIGURE 1. Vacuum Ultrafiltration

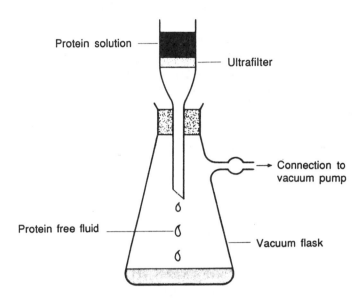

The driving force for the removal of water and dissolved salts by ultrafiltration is the blood pressure prevailing within the capillaries. This pressure overcomes the force which tends to retain fluid within the circulation, namely the colloid osmotic pressure of the blood proteins[13]. In that segment of a capillary immediately following the terminal portion of the smallest artery - the precapillary arteriole of the so-called arterial segment of the loop - the blood pressure is somewhat higher than colloid osmotic pressure and as a consequence ultrafiltration occurs - an escape of water and solutes into the interstitial fluid. The opposite situation exists in the post-capillary or venous side of the capillary network; here the colloid osmotic pressure is higher than the blood pressure. Consequently ultra-filtration takes place from interstitial tissues into the circulation - a process which we call *absorption* or *reabsorption.*

(13) The concentration of blood proteins normally amounts to 7g / 100 ml

It was not without reason that we stated that the capillary walls are *for the most part* impermeable to dissolved proteins. Indeed they are not *completely* impermeable. *A fraction of the blood proteins does actually leave the blood circulating in the capillary bed* - a fact which is of major importance for the subject of this handbook and which will guide us on our way like a golden thread.

As a consequence of the escape of protein through the capillary wall, the interstitial fluid invariably contains some protein. Each protein molecule leaving the blood circulation reduces the colloid osmotic pressure within the terminal vessels, as we will see. We are accustomed to speak, therefore, of an "effective" - that is a practical - colloid osmotic pressure whenever we discuss questions of water and solute exchange between blood and interstitial tissues through the capillary wall:

Effective colloid osmotic pressure =

colloid osmotic pressure within the blood

- colloid osmotic pressure in the interstitial fluid

One further complicating factor is the pressure within the interstitial tissues. It is readily appreciated that this pressure has a similar influence on effective ultrafiltration pressure, just as the colloid osmotic pressure of tissue fluids influences effective colloid osmotic pressure.

Effective ultra-filtration pressure =

blood pressure within the capillaries

- interstitial pressure

We have intentionally avoided giving measurable values to the different pressures under discussion. To do this and to introduce a mathematical formula one would easily be tempted to invoke a series of mathematical calculations. This is done repeatedly in the technical literature only to arrive at fallacious deductions. The pressure in the arterial and venous vascular bed cannot be stated except as an average reading. The pressure falls from the arterial to the venous side of the capillary bed and is influenced by the requirements of the perfused tissues prevailing at the time. If one accepts a figure for intra-capillary pressure, it would only be a statistical average. As a result of water loss through the capillary wall, the protein concentration gradually rises from the arterial to the venous side of the capillary network. It is also misleading to calculate the protein content of a venous blood sample and consider this figure to be identical with the protein content of the capillary blood. Interstitial pressure is not known with certainty. It is sufficient to say in this regard that there are several "interstitial pressures". Thus there is a level of pressure prevailing in the "prelymphatic tissue canals" and in these the tissue fluid lies free. It is accepted today that the pressure here is negative, that is subatmospheric. There is also a pressure within the ground substance of connective tissue and this pressure is positive. The colloid osmotic pressure of interstitial fluid is not identical with that of the interstitial tissue as a whole, nor can it be measured accurately.

Ultrafiltration and reabsorption are naturally determined in like manner by the nature, that is the degree of permeabillity, of the capillary wall for water and protein. This varies in the different segments of the capillary circulation and from organ to organ. One further complicating factor, as already mentioned, is that capillary circulation is by no means constant. In fact, in some individual capillaries circulation is entirely in abeyance. Naturally then, there is neither ultrafiltration nor reabsorption. Because of this we say that one of the factors influencing ultrafiltration or reabsorption is the surface area of the capillary bed actually being perfused.

That part of the interstitial fluid which fails to find its way into the circulation by reabsorption reaches the lymphatics by way of the system of prelymphatic canals[14].

The uptake of interstitial fluid by pores in the lymphatic wall is a complicated process, the exact mechanism of which is still debated in scientific circles today. It involves the normal structure of the

(14) prelymphatic - situated before or proximal to the lymphatic

25

interstitial tissue and the lymphatic capillary. Within the lymphatic the composition of interstitial fluid may change; in general it becomes more concentrated. In contradistinction to the fluid passing through the prelymphatic canals, the fluid contained within the capillary lumen is already identifiable as lymph.

In healthy adults, one to two litres of lymph reaches the circulation by way of the thoracic duct during the course of a day. If one compares the quantity of liquid within the total blood compartment moved by the heart through the blood vessels (this amounts to 10,000 litres in one day) then this two litre quantity appears insignificant. Just the same, these two litres are important to life. The protein content of the thoracic duct lymph is approximately 4%. This means that we are dealing with an appreciable amount of protein. Under conditions of illness, lymph flow can exceed its normal volume twenty fold. The so-called "safety valve function" of the lymphatic apparatus is a very important facility. We will have to go into this matter more fully, because by its safety valve function the lymphatic system ensures that the body is protected against the development of oedema and at the same time - through transport back into the circulation - it prevents (or at least delays) circulatory collapse resulting from an "empty heart beat".

2. OEDEMA AS A SYMPTOM

Before we discuss the safety valve function of the lymphatic system we should explain the meaning of the word "oedema"[1]. By oedema we mean a visible and palpable swelling of some part of the body, i.e. something appreciated by our sense organs, which results from the accumulation of free fluid in the interstitial tissues. Oedema is not a disease but a symptom, one which is associated with a variety of illnesses.

The safety valve function of the lymphatic system is always invoked when the normal balance between the forces of ultrafiltration and reabsorption in the terminal circulation swings in favour of ultrafiltration. This condition arises whenever:

1) the effective ultrafiltration pressure rises;

2) the colloid osmotic pressure falls.

It is understandable that a simultaneous rise in blood pressure in the terminal circulation and a fall in the protein concentration of the blood act in concert, that is in an additive manner.

If we add an increase in permeability to protein of the capillary wall - this is the situation in acute infection - then the lymphatic system intervenes with its safety valve function.

2.1 Oedema as a consequence of "dynamic decompensation" of the lymphatic system.

An example of increased pressure in the terminal circulation occurs typically in people suffering from chronic venous insufficiency. In those, for example, who have suffered from venous thrombosis in the leg, one result can be failure of the valves of the leg veins, with the result that when adopting the upright posture an alteration of venous blood flow takes place, leading to an increase in pressure in the blood capillaries. Ultrafiltration now gains the upper hand over

(1) Greek: oidao - swelling

reabsorption resulting in flooding of the interstitial tissues with fluid. The lymphatic system reacts at once - lymphatic flow increases to a marked degree and fluid is drained from the interstitial tissues. Through its safety valve function, the onset of oedema has been prevented. The function of any organ is naturally limited by its ability to respond to challenge. We can lift up only a certain weight, we can run only at a certain speed for a limited time etc. The volume of fluid which can be taken up in a certain time from the prelymphatic canals through the lymph capillaries and then transported through the lymphatics likewise has an upper limit. This upper limit is termed the *"transport capacity of the lymphatic system"* (Figure 2).

Only when the flow of liquid in unit time from capillaries to tissue fluid - the *lymphatic workload* - exceeds the transport capacity of the lymphatic system will fluid begin to dam up and oedema result. The condition in which the healthy lymphatic system, in spite of summoning up its maximum transport capacity, is unable to cope with the enormous load required of it is spoken of as *"dynamic decompensation"* of the lymphatic system. We are now dealing with *"high volume failure"*, that is decompensation in the presence of greatly increased lymph flow.

The equilibrium which exists between effective filtration pressure and effective colloid osmotic pressure normally present can also be upset by a situation in which effective colloid osmotic pressure falls.

There are kidney diseases ("the nephrotic syndrome") in which the kidneys continually excrete large amounts of protein in the urine. The liver - the factory for circulating blood proteins - actually increases production of new proteins. Because, however, this organ also has a limited production capacity, a fall in plasma proteins will gradually occur. Ultrafiltration from the blood capillaries will now gain the ascendency, thereby prompting the lymphatic system to respond by increasing lymphatic flow and thus preventing oedema formation. *It is only when the situation has reached such great proportions that the volume of fluid flowing out in unit time exceeds*

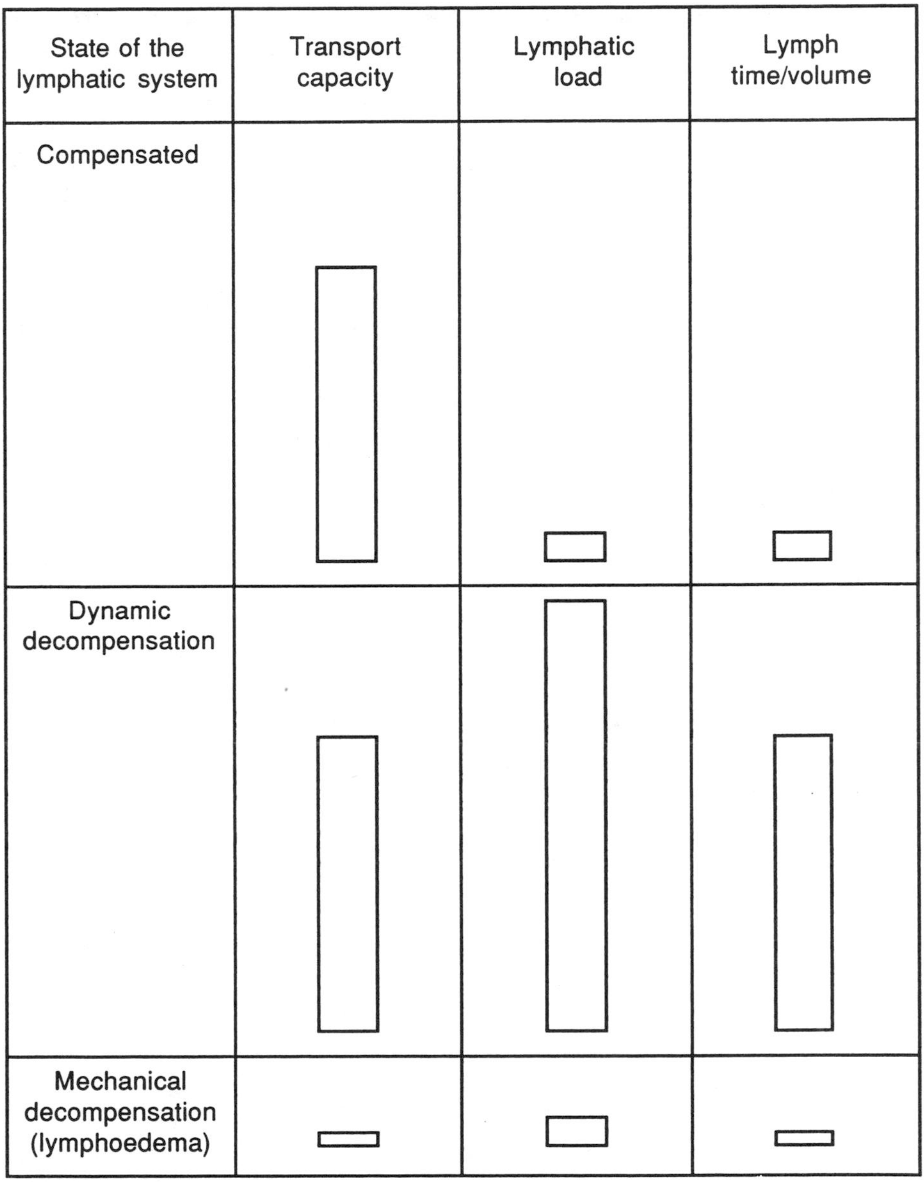

State of the lymphatic system	Transport capacity	Lymphatic load	Lymph time/volume
Compensated			
Dynamic decompensation			
Mechanical decompensation (lymphoedema)			

FIGURE 2. Lymphatic load, transport capacity of the lymphatic system and volume of lymph per unit time under normal conditions, in dynamic high volume decompensation and in lymphoedema (low volume decompensation).

the capacity of the lymphatic system to carry it away will it lead to the accumulation of fluid which we call oedema.

The same situation can arise when the body continually loses protein, not through the kidneys but from the intestines. What particularly interests us here is a disturbance of the intrinsic lymphatics of the bowel wall which leads to local lymphoedema. In this illness, the *lymphostatic* form of the so-called "protein losing enteropathy"[2], protein continually seeps through the oedematous bowel wall and is lost to the body in the faeces. The result is a fall in blood protein concentration. In this way a pathological change, confined initially to the intestinal wall, leads secondarily to generalised oedema. This picture is very easily confused with the more commonly seen kidney complaint, the so-called nephrotic syndrome, which is marked by a similar generalised oedema. The difference is simply that, in the case of protein losing enteropathy, protein cannot be detected in the urine.

A similar mechanism is found in famine oedema. Here the raw materials from which the chemical factory, the liver, manufactures blood proteins are lacking. It is not surprising, therefore, that the end result is a lack of blood proteins. A serious complication arises in famine oedema when there is wasting of body tissues combined with vitamin deficiency and unrestricted intake of salt and water, as salt acts to retain water.

Inflammatory processes are marked by increased permeability of capillaries with respect to blood proteins. The situation can easily arise in which the protein load imposed on the capillaries suddenly increases to such a degree that the healthy lymphatic system cannot keep pace with it. Inflammatory oedema is the consequence of dynamic decompensation. (If the inflammatory process also involves the lymphatics, the transport capacity of the damaged lymphatic system also falls. The "safety valve" function of the lymphatic system soon breaks down with even more devastating consequences (more later).

(2) enteropathy = intestinal disease

In describing the origin of these forms of oedema, our aim naturally enough is not to give a comprehensive survey of the entire problem. Oedema formation is in reality much more complicated. In every individual case of oedema formation many additional mechanisms play a part but have been glossed over intentionally. It suffices here merely to mention that *inadequacy of the lymphatic system is integral to the development of oedema.*

To summarize what has been said already: *In dynamic decompensation of the lymphatic system, the system itself is healthy. It continues to function under the influence of the sheer force of the musculature of the lymphangion to the limit of its transport capacity.* It is not surprising that, after a certain time, the musculature exhibits evidence of fatigue. This then leads to a fall in transport capacity of the lymphatic system. Faced with an ever increasing workload the lymphatics inevitably must fail, leading to increasing oedema.

2.2 "Mechanical decompensation" of the lymphatic system and its consequences. Lymphostatic oedema - the disease known as lymphoedema

It is quite another matter when the lymphatic workload is normal but the lymphatics are defective so that their transport capacity is reduced to such a degree that the normally occurring protein load can no longer be removed. This is termed *"low volume failure"*. It is easily understood that, when the transport capacity of the lymphatic system is reduced under normal conditions of protein load, oedema must develop. We are speaking now of *"mechanical failure"* of the lymphatic system as a consequence of which *"lymphostatic oedema"* or *"lymphoedema"* has occurred. We will examine thoroughly the means by which disease of the lymphatics plays its part.

The normal interstitial tissue can be likened to an alpine meadow traversed by a rippling, crystal-clear brook. The oedema of dynamic failure of the lymphatic system resembles the situation after heavy rainfall followed by brimming banks and flooding of the meadow. On the other hand, the situation found in lymphostasis resembles an evil smelling swamp. Lymphostasis compromises supply and disposal in the tissues, not only through increased space between capillary and cell and increased pressure within the interstitial tissues, but also as a result of slowing down the *"extravascular circulation"* of blood proteins. The body reacts to this situation, which resembles an injury, by increasing "proliferation" and/or fat deposition. To supply this new tissue an entire network of blood vessels is formed. This means that, after a certain time, the "visible and palpable swelling" is not only due to accumulation of water or solutes in the interstitial tissues.

Our therapeutic measures are directed towards the removal of dammed up water and dissolved substances, particularly protein. With lymphatic oedema, still dependent on water and protein held back in the tissues, complete return to normal can be achieved by COMBINED PHYSICAL THERAPY expertly performed: the volume of the affected limb can approximate to that of the healthy one. If connective tissue and/or fat has already been laid down, there remains by the end of phase one of treatment a volume surplus equivalent to this new tissue. In drawing this conclusion, we need say no more than to add that treatment for this oedema should be instituted as soon as possible.

It is to be regretted that many doctors hold the opinion that lymphoedema of modest degree (e.g. a difference of two to five centimetres in the girth of the oedematous arm following surgery or radiotherapy for breast cancer) does not require treatment. Still more regrettable is the notion, often put forward without reservation, that lymphoedema must be accepted simply as a misfortune. One of the patients admitted to our clinic with an extreme degree of lymphatic elephantiasis told us that the doctor whom she had consulted twenty years earlier, when she was in the early stages of lymphoedema, had said: "Many people have blue eyes, many are bald, others have lymphoedema. Nothing can be done for blue eyes, thinning hair or lymphoedema". To establish the diagnosis, he proceeded to lymphangiography and then left the patient to her fate. Thereupon she did precisely nothing for two decades. (Figure 3)

Chronic lymph stasis has been recognized as bearing a strong relationship to infection. According to Professor *Brunner's* studies,

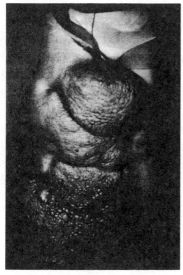
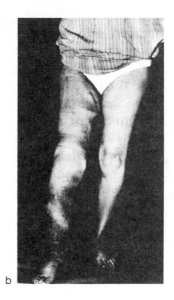

a b

FIGURE 3:

(a) Lymphostatic elephantiasis in a 38 year old woman before treatment. Onset of lymphoedema at the age of 18 years. She remained untreated for 20 years, and her condition progressively deteriorated. The circumference of the thigh measured 118 cm. The patient was unable to walk, and sexual activity had been impossible for some time. There was severe inflammation with high fever and raised sedimentation rate.

(b) With appropriate medical treatment followed by Complex Physical Therapy (CPT), the elephantiasis was considerably improved. Assisted by "phase 2 of maintaining and maximizing" by CPT, the condition was permanently controlled. The patient was once again able to work.

fungal infections of the foot are found about three times more commonly in oedematous legs than in the healthy control group. The fungal infections, evidenced by severe itching and burning between the toes, lead to cracks in the skin which act as a portal of entry for various bacteria such as streptococci and often staphylococci. These bring about a dreaded complication of lymphoedema, namely erysipelas. As we have described, this inflammatory process is accompanied by increased capillary permeability. This in turn increases workload in a situation where the transport capacity of the lymphatics is already greatly reduced. Naturally this must lead to worsening of the lymphoedema. Extravasated blood proteins, along with the debris of dead cells, clog the tissues and perpetuate the vicious cycle of inflammation. When this also involves the lymphatics, their functional state, and hence their transport capacity, is still further reduced. Weakness, even paralysis or spastic contraction of the capillary wall can result. All of these encourage lymph stasis. Erysipelas must inevitably lead to deterioration of lymphoedema. Table 3 sets out these relationships and the vicious cycle which has, as its end point, worsening of the chronic lymphoedema.

TABLE 3. The vicious cycle of inflammation and lymphoedema.

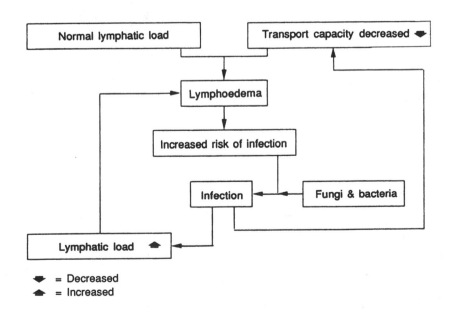

To the physician, an understanding of these relationships is of practical importance, not to be underrated. Only the doctor who is aware of these can correctly advise his patient about lymphoedema, and only the patient able to appreciate the wisdom of the various injunctions restricting lifestyle (tables 6 and 7) will carry out these instructions to the letter.

The problems of inflammation lead us at once to the third and main type of decompensation of the lymphatic system, that of the failure of its *safety valve function*. It appears that the carrying capacity of the lymphatic system in severe lymphoedema is greatly depressed, and at the same time the workload increased to such a degree that it must exceed even the great transport capacity of a *normal* lymphatic system. In such cases we see no ordinary lymphoedema, but extensive cell damage from severe water-logging of the tissues. At this stage, we will not concern ourselves further with these interesting and important questions.

3. CLASSIFICATION OF LYMPHOEDEMA

It is common practice in medicine to use the term *secondary* when the cause of an illness is known with certainty and *primary* when this is not the case. In classifying the various forms of lymphoedema we have adopted this practice.

3.1 Primary lymphoedema

One of the great marvels of creation is the fact that the fertilised egg contains all the information necessary for a human being to be born into the world nine months later, crafted according to an exact predetermined plan, and imbued with normal function. Considering the amazing complexity of development, it is surprising therefore that developmental abnormalities occur so rarely, and it is the greater wonder that development almost always proceeds according to plan.

Abnormalities of all the organs and organ systems are well known. It is no surprise therefore that they can also arise in the developing lymphatic system. The most serious defects of the lymphatic system, which result in complete failure of lymph flow, are incompatible with life. The embryo, monstrously bloated by severe oedema, dies in the womb.

According to our present day knowledge, primary lymphoedema arises as a result of developmental abnormalities. The lymph vessels are either too few in number and too finely constructed *(hypoplasia)*$_{(1)}$ or there is *hyperplasia*$_{(2)}$. This can be compared to the marked difference between varicose and normal veins. Insufficiency of the valves may be an associated anomaly. Primary lymphoedema of the leg can also be caused by fibrosis of the inguinal lymph nodes. There are also cases of primary lymphoedema

(1) hypoplasia - underdevelopment

(2) hyperplasia - overdevelopment

based on *aplasia*₍₃₎ of lymph capillaries alongside normal collecting vessels.

Lymphangiectasis can be associated with so-called *chylous reflux*. Normally, lymph rich in fat (chyle) flows from the small intestine into the *cisterna chyli*. This reservoir, lying under the diaphragm and behind the peritoneum (which lines the abdominal cavity), also receives lymphatics from the rest of the intestinal tract, liver and pancreas, kidneys, sex organs and pelvis, and the lower limbs. The thoracic duct arises from the cisterna chyli and, passing through the diaphragm and the posterior part of the thoracic cavity as already described, enters the *vena cava*. After a fatty meal, chyle becomes a turbid, milky fluid. Normally, backflow of lymph and chyle is prevented by a system of functioning valves.

The lymphangiectatic₍₄₎ form of primary lymphoedema, and also chylous obstruction, can lead to valve failure through dilatation of the lymphatics, and this will allow retrograde flow of chyle. After a fatty meal, the turbid milky fluid may escape through so-called lymph fistulas (in the skin, genitalia, renal pelvis, abdominal cavity etc). In this way reflux can occur.

Primary lymphoedema can often be sporadic and familial in its presentation. There are both congenital and acquired forms.

3.1.1 *Primary lymphoedema of insidious onset.*

In most cases, the onset of the acquired form of primary lymphoedema is slow and gradual without any demonstrable causal factor. The following case record is typical: About a year after the onset of menstruation, a young girl develops swelling on the dorsum of one foot. The swelling is painless and skin discoloration is lacking; it is only noticeable because her shoe feels tight. Slowly, over the course of weeks, months or years, the swelling reaches the ankle and lower calf. Initially the swelling is soft, producing at first

---

(3) aplasia (Greek) - an inborn growth defect

(4) lymphangiectasis (Greek ectasis = widening) - pathological dilatation of the lymphatics.

a hollow on finger pressure ("pitting") over the lower tibial bone. This swelling goes away partly or completely with a night's rest. The lymphoedema is in the first or *reversible* stage. Later the swelling will remain even after rest. Because of the slow development of thickening of the tissues, pitting will be produced with difficulty or not at all, and the volume of the limb will slowly increase. In most cases the pitting will be firm. This is then the second or *chronic reversible* stage of lymphoedema.

A transient increase in swelling in both the reversible and the irreversible stages may be provoked by prolonged standing, sitting or exposure to heat. There is occasionally a premenstrual increase. *Stemmer* has described an unusual but characteristic sign in lymphoedema - induration and loss of flexibility of the skin creases. A later development is the so-called lymphostatic hyperkeratosis[5] (Fig. 4, 5).

When lymph stasis is present, it is not unusual for mycotic infection or cellulitis to affect the limb and lead to dramatic worsening of the complaint. Pregnancy may also lead to progression into the *third stage of lymphatic elephantiasis*. According to studies by Professor *Brunner,* one can anticipate that lymphoedema will deteriorate after the third pregnancy. Unwarranted and invasive diagnostic measures, and/or an incorrect treatment regimen, could also lead to deterioration or more rapid progression.

Lymphostatic elephantiasis was described in 1892 by *Winiwarter* as follows:

> "Through increasing swelling the girth of the limb reaches monstrous proportions. The leg, in particular, resembles a misshapen, uniformly thickened cylinder "like pantaloons" gathered at the ankle, below which the foot is much smaller in size, or from which thick rolls or flaps hang down over the instep or the sides of the foot, reaching the floor like folds of a garment, while the foot itself retains normal dimensions. However if the elephantiasis has involved the foot, it comes to resemble a shapeless blob..."

(5) *Lymphostatic hyperkeratosis = extremely dense induration of the skin with the development of calluses and wart-like projections, due to lymph stasis.*

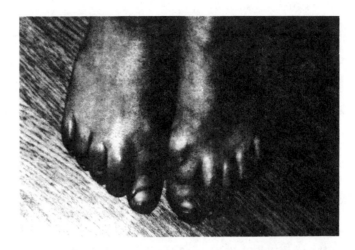

FIGURE 4. Primary lymphoedema of the right foot. Positive "Stemmer's sign": paucity and rigidity of skin folds around the toes.

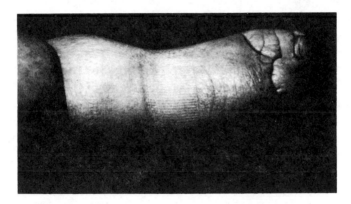

FIGURE 5. "Lymphostatic hyperkeratosis" in a patient with primary lymphoedema of the leg. Oedematous instep and deep, dimpled crease at the level of the ankle.

Should the onset of lymphoedema be before the age of 35, it is termed *lymphoedema praecox*[6]. If the disease first starts after 35 it is termed *lymphoedema tardum*[7]. The inherited form is known as *lymphoedema congenitum*.

(6) *praecox = premature*

(7) *tardus/a/um = late or slow.*

It should be pointed out at this juncture that the diagnosis of primary lymphoedema, especially lymphoedema tardum, can only be made when a diligent search has been undertaken to rule out lymphoedema secondary to malignant disease.

Many doctors find it puzzling that *hereditary* lymphangiopathy[8] never develops into hereditary lymphoedema; the latter may appear only after decades, as we have seen.

The explanation is simple. In spite of the inherited abnormality, the transport capacity of the lymphatic system, although limited from the point of view of its functional reserve, can deal with a *normal* lymphatic workload. It only reaches the point of *lymphangiopathy with an incompetent lymphatic system* (in other words to lymphoedema) when the transport capacity of the lymphatic system falls still further and can no longer handle a normal lymphatic workload. This may result from fatigue of the lymphangion after many years of over-distension of its musculature. It becomes weak, and passive dilatation of the lymphatic ensues. The valves can no longer close, and lymph flow comes to a standstill. The end result is then an overtaxed lymphatic wall initially saturated with lymph, that is with a protein-rich fluid. A later result is proliferation of connective tissue with still greater reduction of its ability to contract. Finally the lymphatic becomes a rigid, immobile tube. Of course, stiffening of the lymphatic wall through age plays an additional role. An even worse situation occurs if for any reason there is increased workload. Trivial injury, possibly unnoticed at the time, or fungal infection is sufficient to bring this about.

3.1.2 *Primary lymphoedema of sudden onset*

In contradistinction to the type of primary oedema already mentioned, this complaint is occasionally sudden in onset, occurring out of the blue. Sometimes a precipitating factor such as injury can be identified, but in many cases there is none. The following case history is typical of *post-traumatic[9] primary lymphoedema:* A

(8) *disease of lymphatic vessels*

(9) *following injury*

young woman sprains her foot; the ankle swells. The swelling does not subside but involves the instep, then gradually spreads to the calf and later the thigh. Often an orthopaedic surgeon is consulted early in the illness. An Unnas stocking is applied but must soon be removed because of intolerable pressure symptoms. The swelling persists, and from that time on proceeds inexorably. This is described in detail on pages 37 and 38 from the initial reversible stage to the third stage, that of elephantiasis, similar to cases of primary lymphoedema of insidious onset. (It should be mentioned here that, as well as post-traumatic primary lymphoedema, there is also a post-traumatic seconday form - see page 43).

An insect bite or an infection (fungal, erysipeloid) can similarly lead to the sudden appearance of primary lymphoedema. The explanation for primary lymphoedema after trivial injury is simple. The delicate balance between normal lymphatic workload and that which prevails with drastically impaired lymph transport capacity due to congenital lymphangiopathy means that a mere cut or inflammatory lesion is enough to increase this burden. At the same time however, lymphatics are severed or blocked by lymphangitis as the case may be. The equilibrium is upset and the end result is an accumulation of protein material in the interstitial tissues and lymphoedema (table 4). Often no explanation can be found (table 5).

Primary lymphoedema can be unilateral at first - the other limb can swell up in the same way even years later. There are also cases in which the disease remains unilateral throughout life. We know from lymphangiographic studies that, in these cases, the leg which is free of oedema remains in a state of *lymphangiopathy with (as yet) adequate lymphatic circulation*. Based on arguments presented already, this situation is understandable.

3.1.3. Primary lymphoedema and other developmental abnormalities

Primary lymphoedema can be associated with other developmental abnormalities, alone or in combination. For example a heart defect, congenital dislocation of the hip, spina bifida, congenital fusion of the fingers, supranumerary fingers and/or toes, hare lip and cleft

TABLE 4. In the case of lymphangiopathy with inadequate lymphatic function, an injury of only minor degree suffices to bring about decompensation and hence lymphoedema.

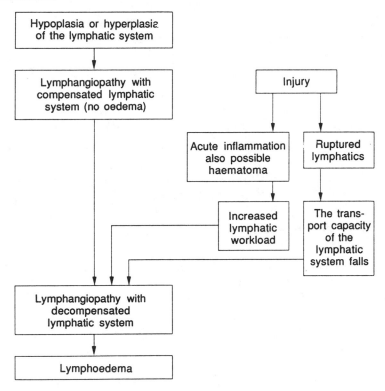

palate etc. The *yellow fingernail syndrome*[10] consists of a triad[11] of dystrophic[12] fingernails, oedematous limbs and pleuro-pulmonary lymphangiopathy. The association of primary lymphoedema with lymphatic enteropathy[13] is of importance. This is a special form of *protein-losing enteropathy,* whereby lymphatic oedema of the wall of the small intestine may or may not lead to reflux of chyle into the bowel lumen. The net result is protein loss in the stools.

(10) syndrome: a symptom complex or group of physical signs appearing together.

(11) triad: a syndrome with three components.

(12) dystrophy: disturbance of growth or nutrition.

(13) enteropathy: a bowel disorder or defect.

TABLE 5. In cases of lymphangiopathy with a still adequate lymphatic system, gradual "fatigue" of the overloaded lymphatics, or ageing changes, may result in chronc lymphoedema.

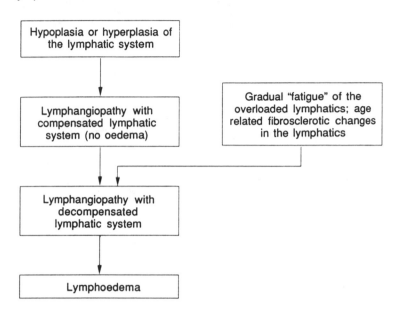

When this protein loss exceeds the ability of the liver to manufacture more protein, the plasma protein concentration falls and hypoproteinaemic[14] oedema results.

3.2 Secondary lymphoedema

We speak of secondary lymphoedema when the cause of the lymphangiopathy which leads to low volume failure of the lymphatic system is known. Injury, lymphangitis, surgical intervention, malignant disease or self-mutilation may be the cause of mechanical decompensation of the lymphatic system resulting in secondary lymphoedema.

In patients with lymphangiopathy but a still adequate lymphatic system, a trivial injury is enough to trigger post-traumatic primary lymphoedema. In contrast, patients with a normally developed lymphatic system require the severest injury - as for example

(14) *hypoproteinaemic: lowered concentration of plasma proteins.*

extensive skin abrasions where normal regeneration of lymphatics is prevented by scar formation and thus progresses to post-traumatic lymphoedema. It is part of the varied response of the body that, after extensive severance of lymphatics, they will soon regenerate. Hence the body has four options:

1) The surviving lymphatics dilate and form a *collateral circulation;*

2) new anastomoses$_{(15)}$ develop between proximal and distal ends of the severed vessels: *"interlymphatic anastomoses"*

3) the lymphatics drain into veins: *"lymph-venous anastomoses"*;

4) the obstructed site is by-passed by dilated *prelymphatic channels.*

In this way a compensatory mechanism is brought about, dependent on the lymphatic system. Dwindling lymph flow encourages the migration of monocytes $_{(16)}$ from blood capillaries into the potentially lymphoedematous area where they are transformed into macrophages$_{(17)}$. These engulf proteins trapped in the area of stasis, and thus diminish the protein load which must be cleared away. Lymphoedema now develops only if there is failure of lymphatic regeneration as well as macrophage activity. Secondary lymphoedema can be a consequence of inflammation of lymphatics (lymphangitis) regardless of whether the inflammation is due to bacteria, fungi, parasites, insect bites or foreign particulate matter. In tropical countries many millions suffer from lymphoedema due to the parasitic disease filariasis. In Ethiopia, dust rich in silica penetrates the soles of those walking barefoot and thereby rendered more vulnerable to injury. This produces lymphangitis and permanent lymphatic obstruction.

Under "iatrogenic forms" is implied lymphoedema *secondary to medical* treatment. There are two distinctly different types. In the

(15) anastomosis: tributaries or connections between two vessels.

(16) monocyte: a type of white blood corpuscle

(17) macrophage: a large scavenger cell

first instance, the doctor is obliged to block lymph drainage from part of the body and accept lymphoedema as a consequence when the procedure in question is a necessary and justifiable, but unavoidable, part of the treatment of malignant disease. Cancer cells have the ability to invade the lymphatic system from their site of origin and to form metastatic[18] deposits in the regional lymph nodes. This will be discussed in greater detail in the chapter on secondary lymphoedema of the upper limb after surgery and radiotherapy for cancer of the breast. In the second instance, lymphoedema may be the unfortunate consequence of unskilled medical treatment. Even removal of a segment of vein for use in a by-pass operation can lead to iatrogenic lymphoedema of the leg, and nobody should blame the vascular surgeon for this. On the other hand, unskilful medical and surgical procedures will occasionally cause lymphoedema.

The following however is important. In the case of groin surgery the greatest care must be exercised, both in the decision to operate and in the operation itself. All the lymphatics from the lower limb come together at this site. A broad, horizontal incision can sever the entire lymph drainage from the leg and, at the same time, block lymphatic drainage from the external genitalia. A basic rule is therefore: avoid surgical removal of fatty or fibrous tumours from the groin! Cautious removal of groin lymph nodes for histological examination is permissible, but only when requested by an experienced oncologist[19]. (In cases of malignant disease the guidelines are of course well defined; the whole groin area must be cleared and the possibility of lymphoedema accepted). The popliteal space[20] is a particularly risky site as the lymphatic drainage from the leg and foot comes together behind the knee. We continue to see patients in whom fatty deposits have been cleared from the popliteal space, and the end result of this unnecessary surgery can be iatrogenic lymphoedema of the leg and foot. Special care is required after operations on the knee cartilages.

(18) metastasis (Greek): distant secondary deposit.

(19) oncologist: a specialist in malignant disease

(20) popliteal space: the hollow behind the knee.

By "stripping" is understood operative removal of varicose veins. If this procedure is carried out expertly, the lymph collecting tubes lying adjacent to the veins can be spared. An unskilled operator can easily damage lymphatics and cause lymphoedema. In expert hands, lymphoedema will follow arterial reconstruction surgery in only 2% of cases. People who seek vascular surgery on purely cosmetic grounds should be mindful of this fact. *"Post reconstructive"* or *"post ischaemic"* lymphoedema can arise as a serious complication of restorative operations for the treatment of arterial disease.

So-called "factitious" lymphoedema can be brought about by self-mutilation. Here is a typical illustrative case history. A young girl was admitted to a paediatric clinic for the diagnosis and investigation of swelling of the instep, ankle and leg. Following extensive investigation, she was discharged with the diagnosis of "idiopathic oedema"$_{(21)}$. Because her condition deteriorated, she was referred to our clinic. A circular line of demarcation, with swelling starting only below this line, permitted a spot diagnosis, later to be confirmed as she was discovered in the toilet applying an elastic band to her leg.

In the management of a case such as this, a psychological approach and sympathetic understanding are required. In the case illustrated, the child's parents were constantly bickering and the father was a chronic alcoholic. The girl was brought up by her grandmother who, after breast surgery, developed secondary oedema of the arm and died soon afterwards of secondary tumour growth. The child identified with the only person who had offered her love and affection. Many cases of artifical oedema can be blamed on economic problems in the family.

The three stages: 1) reversible,

2) spontaneous and irreversible and

3) elephantiasis, are found in secondary just as in primary lymphoedema.
(See pages 37-38)

(21) *oedema of unknown cause.*

3.3 Benign and malignant lymphoedema

The distinction beween malignant[22] and benign lymphoedema is of major importance in diagnosis and treatment. In malignant oedema, the lymph flow is obstructed by malignant disease of any type. It may be the result of a hitherto undiagnosed tumour, or a recurrence of malignant disease following surgery or radiotherapy. Sarcoma and malignant lymphoma can also cause malignant oedema. All other forms of oedema belong to the benign group. *Once the doctor has diagnosed "lymphoedema", it is of paramount importance in medical management to ascertain whether one is dealing with the benign or the malignant form. In other words, an aetiological[23] diagnosis is essential.*

To answer this question the doctor, on principle, must proceed step by step, moving in turn from harmless, non-invasive diagnostic tests to the more invasive[24] ones. A detailed history is of primary importance. This is followed by a complete physical examination, then the necessary laboratory investigations. Sometimes consultation with other specialists is required (haematologist, gynaecologist, urologist, radiologist). Should suspicion fall on a possible malignancy, and histological examination be required, a fine needle biopsy or removal of tissue for examination may be required to further the diagnosis.

Lymphangiography, by direct injection of an oil-based contrast medium, may also be required, *but only as a last resort.* One should never start investigation with lymphangiography. It is not the radiologist's task to recommend gynaecological or urological *examination* after he has performed the *lymphangiogram,* but more correctly *they* should request lymphangiography. Apart from searching for a tumour, lymphangiography for lymphoedema involving a limb is only of academic or historical interest. No lymphangiographic finding influences future management, and the

(22) *In this context "malignant" refers to tumour growth such as cancer.*

(23) *aetiology: the study of cause*

(24) *Invasive: using force, or by penetration of body tissues*

performance of lymphangiography can worsen the situation dramatically[25]. One exception is lymphoedema starting with lymph or chyle reflux. The lymphangiographic finding can influence the *plan of operative treatment* drawn up by a surgeon with special experience in this field.

Imaging by *radio-isotopes* is completely harmless and often rewarding.

This involves injection of a radioactive substance with an affinity for the lymphatic system. The speed with which it is taken up and transported from the injection site to its appearance in the regional lymph nodes can give information about both lymphatic vessels and lymph nodes (Fig. 7).

3.4 Staged classification of lymphoedema

On pages *37-38* and *46* it was stated that, according to Brunner (modified), all types of lymphoedema can be divided into three stages. We call the first the *"reversible stage"*. By this term we mean lymphoedema which disappears with bed rest after a few days, or even overnight. The swelling is soft at this stage, and it will pit easily with light finger pressure. This is due to the fact that, at this early stage, the swelling consists entirely of protein-rich fluid lying in the interstitial tissues. Inevitably however this lymphoedema progresses, sooner or later, to the second stage called the *"spontaneous irreversible stage"*. The situation now is that even a longer period of bed rest will not see the disappearance of the oedema, and the swelling becomes harder. Strong pressure of the finger tip is now required to produce a hollow, or pitting does not appear at all. This stage depends on the slow formation of fibrous tissue (fibrosis) in the area where stasis of protein-rich fluid has occurred. With the passage of time, the newly formed fibrous tissue becomes harder and harder (induration, sclerosis).

(25) *Removal of a segment of lymphangion for histological examination, recommended at one time, has since been shown to be misleading. There is no correlation between clinical and histological findings. In any case, histological examination of lymphoedematous tissue is superfluous. If malignancy is suspected, it can only be used if the doctor cannot arrive at the answer by non-invasive methods.*

As a result of inflammatory insults (these may be caused by bacteria or fungi, or be non-infective), the "spontaneous irreversible stage" passes gradually into the stage of so-called "elephantiasis". This is caused by an extreme degree of swelling of the limb, with thickening of the skin and the production of wart-like excrescences (Fig. 3a).

Long standing elephantiasis carries the risk of a fatal outcome because the highly malignant tumour known as lymphangiosarcoma may develop in the altered tissues.

4. LYMPHOEDEMA OF THE ARM FOLLOWING TREATMENT FOR BREAST CANCER

4.1 *Introduction*

Breast cancer is perceived by any woman as a cruel blow of fate[1]. She must undergo disfiguring surgery to save her life, and to be able to overcome this mentally and physically requires extraordinary strength of will. Immediately after operation or radiotherapy, permanent swelling of the arm can appear - a complication about which the patient is rarely forewarned. In other cases months, years or even several years may elapse. The patient may already have grown accustomed to the loss of a breast - frequently, only the closest family members know about it - then swelling of the arm and perhaps the hand appears. The secret must now be revealed. This visible evidence often leads to more problems than the physical disability which accompanies it. Despairingly the patient asks the question over and over again: "Why must I of all people suffer not only a cancer operation but this second horrible affliction as well? I know many people who have undergone cancer surgery and are left with a normal arm".

The patient now seeks the advice of the oncologist and very often experiences great disappointment. All doctors involved with breast cancer - surgeons, gynaecologists, radiologists - give of their best endeavour. Generally the after-treatment of cancer is well organized in the Federal Republic of Germany. Just the same, the woman suffering from an oedematous arm who looks for help is consoled with the statement: "You can do nothing about it, you just have to *get used to it*". Two fundamental factors underlie this attitude. Unfortunately, doctors *do not know* how to manage an oedematous arm following breast surgery because lymphology is not taught in universities. The other factor has a psychological basis. The patient's life was saved - the price paid for this is trivial - a swollen arm, which must be accepted. Many surgeons are not prepared to accept that a woman on whom they have operated could be left with

---

(1) *Breast cancer seldom occurs in a man, and lymphoedema can follow either surgery or radiotherapy.*

an oedematous arm. "I am a clean and skilful operator - that does not happen to my patients". This is perhaps the main reason why, in medical literature, the frequency of the occurrence of lymphoedema after surgery or radiotherapy is variable, ranging from single figure percentages to over 50%. The only reliable investigation, world-wide, was carried out by Professor Göltner of Fulda who showed that lymphoedema occurs in about 40% of cases. According to *Barth* "the mid-arm circumference after operation, compared to the other side is *almost always* two to five centimetres greater. It leads to no disability and is of no consequence".

In our opinion insignificant swelling never exists. We must guard against it in the early stages and give adequate treatment to overcome it (see below). A patient with an oedematous arm after surgery for breast cancer should not take her problems to an oncologist. *She needs after-treatment for cancer by a lymphologist.* On the other hand, the oncologist's duty should be to make clear to the patient immediately before surgery or radiotherapy that she may develop lymphoedema, and to instruct her on a few rules of conduct which will serve to guard against its development (Table 6).

We reached a similar conclusion in our 1987 published study, which showed an incidence of only 18%. Many oncologists are hardly aware of the problem. Others who know about it adopt the misguided attitude that such a statement would unnecessarily upset a patient already prepared to undergo surgery for breast cancer. We can refute this argument, having found that 97% of the patients whose opinion we sought thought that an explanation was of value. Our opinion is that it is the oncologist's duty to inform the patient in advance of the possible occurrence of secondary lymphoedema of the arm, and impart to her the necessary knowledge so that she will be in a better position to avoid its occurrence.

The measures which have to be adopted in the interest of avoiding a swollen arm add scarcely any burden to the patient's quality of life. We are certain that every woman is thankful for a timely explanation and will readily adopt the measures set out in Table 6. We hear over and over again from patients: "Why was nothing said to me about this? Why was I not told that I could get lymphoedema, or what I should have done to prevent it?" The patient's active co-operation in preventing lymphoedema is mandatory, but it is also essential when lymphoedema is already present. If the patient does not co-operate, even the most skilful medical management is doomed to failure. In our opinion the patient can be motivated to co-operate by an understanding of the normal functioning of the lymphatic system and the nature of the lymphoedema which has given rise to her swollen arm.

TABLE 6. Advice for patients after treatment of breast cancer (surgery, radiotherapy or both) with lymphoedema of the arm.

1. In the home and workplace.
Avoid injury, strain and exposure to heat or cold.

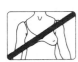
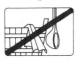

1.1 Careful with that kitchen knife!

1.2 Careful when sewing (use a thimble)!

1.3 Never wash in very hot water.

1.4 Never open or close a window with raised arms.

1.5 Never carry a heavy shopping bag.

1.6 Careful when ironing!

1.7 When you smoke (you should give it up!) do not hold the burning cigarette in the hand at risk.

1.8 Do not wear your watch on the swollen wrist. Always wear your compression stocking when doing housework; for extra protection use rubber gloves.

2. In your dress.

The bra strap should not cut into the shoulder or chest wall. The breast prosthesis should be as light-weight as possible. The sleeves of your dress or blouse should not be too constricting. Skirts or belts should not be too tight - free respiration is important.

3. Cosmetic or beauty treatment, and at the hairdresser.

3.1 In your manicure, do not injure the cuticle.

3.2 Do not use cosmetics which irritate the skin

3.3 No saunas.

3.4 Care when sunbathing - avoid sunburn at all costs!

3.5 No firm arm or trunk massage.

3.6 Protect the shoulder and arm from the heating effect of hairdryers.

4. **In the garden.**
    Avoid injury (spikes, thorns and garden implements)

5. **Cat scratches are to be avoided at all costs!**

6. **In sport.**
    6.1 No backward movement of the shoulder or the swollen arm
        (no tennis or golf!).
    6.2 Beware of frostbite!
    6.3 Avoid injury! (Downhill skiing is dangerous, Nordic skiing
        for practical purposes is safer. Quiet swimming is one of
        the theraputic measures we recommend.)

7. **Diet.**
    7.1 Maintain a sensible weight. In cases of overweight, reduce
        by diet and exercise.
    7.2 Just as there is no "cancer" diet, there is no "lymphoedema"
        diet. Be moderate in your diet.
    7.3 Limit salt intake and take fluids as desired; fluid restric-
        tion is not recommended

8. **Daytime activities.**
    Perform special exercises to reduce swelling. Unless you have
    medical advice to the contrary, do these while wearing the arm
    stocking. Wear a well fitting stocking, one prescribed by the
    doctor.

9. **Before going to bed.**
    Unless otherwise ordered, first careful toilet, then bandage
    your arm.

10. **Planning your holidays.**
    Avoid environments in which insects abound.

11. When visiting the doctor.

11.1 Do not allow your blood pressure to be measured on the affected arm.

11.2 Do not allow any injections (either subcutaneous, intramuscular, intravenous or intra-articular) on the operated side. Do not apply or inject any medication on the operated side.

11.3 Do not allow venepuncture on the operated side.

11.4 No acupuncture treatment, no so-called "Heilanaesthesia" to be carried out on the affected side.

11.5 Do not allow venography or direct lymphography on the swollen arm.

11.6 Never accept manual lymph drainage as the only treatment option. Adequate management implies **Complex Physical Therapy.** Refuse "intermittent compression therapy" or "stripping".

11.7 Never accept a compression stocking without preliminary clearing of the oedema.

12. At the physiotherapist or medical gymnast.

12.1 No firm massage.

12.2 No mud packs on the oedematous limb.

12.3 No electrotherapy to induce deep heat.

12.4 No overzealous medical gymnastics involving the shoulder-joint.

13. VISIT THE DOCTOR AT ONCE:

13.1 If you see signs of inflammation on the swollen arm (reddening of the skin, fever and chills).

13.2 If you see a spot resembling a small haemorrhage on your skin.

13.3 Should pain or muscle weakness occur.

13.4 If the swelling becomes worse in spite of adequate treatment.

4.2 Cause and Extent of Lymphoedema after Surgery or Radiotherapy for Breast Cancer.

Swelling of the arm can appear when only surgery has been performed, even without irradiation. Often both forms of treatment are used. As we have seen, this question is one of secondary lymphoedema. The term "lymphoedema" implies a reduction of transport capacity of the lymphatic system below the normal load threshold. The word "secondary" suggests that it is a consequence of cancer therapy.

Swelling of the arm after cancer surgery or radiotherapy does not depend on obstruction to venous return from the arm to the axillary vein, although unfortunately this view is often erroneously held. This does not mean however that such a condition may not co-exist. It is never the *sole* cause of a swollen arm. If it does occur in isolated cases, it merely increases the severity of the swelling. It is not at all correct to embark on *venography* as a means of investigating the swollen arm, yet this is often recommended by doctors. To perform venography, a radiographic contrast material must be injected into a vein in the bend of the elbow. This diagnostic procedure can lead, in itself, to an increase in the swelling. A corollary to this is that the findings from venography do not influence the choice of therapeutic measures for lymphoedema. Venolysis - freeing of veins in the armpit from constricting fibrous tissue - is not encouraged by lymphologists.

Why does secondary lymphoedema occur in the arm? We know already that cancer cells tend to migrate to regional lymph nodes from the primary nodes close to the seat of the tumour. The important regional lymph nodes in relation to the breast are found in the armpit *(axilla)*. This is the reason why the surgeon must remove not only the affected breast but also the axillary lymph nodes. It is only by histological examination of the excised nodes that one can find out whether they contain metastases. It is true that the arm lymphatics as well as those of the upper region of the trunk on the same side empty into the axillary nodes - if not all, then the majority of them. Through removal of axillary lymph nodes - not only intentional, but necessary, the lymphatic drainage from the arm as well as the adjacent upper quarter of the trunk is inter-rupted (Fig 6). We would stress that this does not imply an error on the surgeon's part, but is an unavoidable part of cancer treatment!

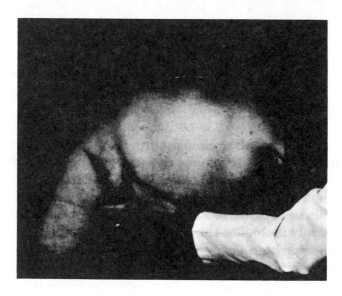

FIGURE 6. Oedema of cutaneous tissues over the ipsilateral upper quadrant of the thorax and increased skinfold thickness.

The course taken by the lymphatics in the arm differs from person to person. There are women whose arm lymphatics drain into the axillary nodes, and there are others in whom an arm lymphatic vessel - we call it the "cephalic$_{(2)}$ vessel" empties into a lymph node which lies above the clavicle or collarbone. One can readily appre-ciate that women endowed with a "cephalic" lymphatic vessel are able to escape lymphoedema of the arm after radical breast sur-gery, or that immediately after the operation swelling appears and then gradually goes away. A pre-requisite for this is that the "cephalic" vessel takes over the function of the missing lymphatics, forms a collateral circulation, and assumes the workload of the arm lymphatics. The situation now arises that it not only drains lymph from the upper ("short cephalic vessel"), but also from the forearm

(2) *Greek: kephalos - head*

56

(the long vessel). A collateral circulation can be established both to the contralateral_(3) as well as the ipsilateral_(4) axilla. There still remains the considerable capacity of the lymphatic system to regenerate (mentioned already). The two severed ends of the vessel can link up again, and by this means the lymph flow to the axilla, interrupted by surgery, can be restored. A proviso, however, is that scar tissue does not form in the depths of the operative field because this prevents the severed vessels from joining up. This means that women lacking a "long cephalic vessel" draining into a supraclavicular node can also remain free of oedema.

The reader must surely have wondered at this stage how a solitary lymphatic vessel (the "cephalic"), having its source outside the axilla, can possibly be in a position to effect drainage from the whole arm, normally carried out by a great number of vessels. How can this one vessel suddenly manage to transport many times its normal lymph flow? Had the lymphatic been an inert channel this would surely not be possible. If, before clearing the axillary nodes, the "cephalic" lymphatic vessel is given all at once the task of taking over the entire workload of the severed lymphatics, this additional work would be only achieved by adaptation to new circumstances. The lymphatics are furnished with a well-developed smooth muscle component whose activity is under nervous control. Lymph flow is maintained by pulsation of this musculature. The valves which occur at regular intervals along the vessel ensure that the lymph flow is directed centrally from the periphery. Whenever workload increases, the vessels dilate and begin to pulsate with greater force and frequency. By this means, the flow of lymph through the vessel in unit time is enormously increased. To achieve this increased workload, the thickness of the muscle fibres within the vessel wall increases, just as limb muscles increase in bulk through training.

Knowledge about these facts is not only of theoretical importance, but has far reaching practical consequences, as it influences in no small measure the lifestyle of a woman who has undergone breast surgery.

(3) *contralateral - on the opposite side*

(4) *ipsilateral - the same side*

Just as in training for sport, when one wishes to achieve a high peak of efficiency, the workload must be increased in a careful and sensible way to avoid over-strain, so the lymphatic musculature must not be exposed to any additional and unnecessary stress. Of course, as already stated, it is also possible for severed axillary lymphatics to regenerate and thereby to fully restore the lymph flow in the arm back to normal. Just the same, we cannot be sure whether we will achieve an oedema free state after surgery or radiotherapy for breast cancer, or whether we will arrive at this happy situation when freedom from oedema, brought about by inadequate axillary lymph flow, will be achievable through greater efforts of adaptation on the part of a "long cephalic vessel".

This question cannot be settled by recourse to lymphography, that is by surgical exposure of a lymphatic in the forearm whereby an oily contrast medium is injected into the vessel. This could result, moreover, in obstruction of the lymphatic by injuring its wall and so lead to lymphoedema.

To be safe, we must accept that we are dealing with a fragile vessel carrying out its task under duress, and spare it. *Tiedjen's* observations are relevant. After surgery and radiotherapy for breast cancer, the removal of radioactive material injected into hand tissues is delayed, even when lymphatic oedema is absent (Fig 7).

The lymphatic workload should under no circumstances exceed the normal, because exhaustion of the lymphatic musculature is an inevitable consequence. If this situation should occur, the muscle will fatigue and the vessel will passively dilate. As a result of this widening, the valves no longer close and lymph flow comes to a halt. Stasis extends from the connecting vessels to the capillaries and these cease their normal activity. Tissue fluid rich in protein clogs up the *prelymphatic canals*, and the pressure rises in lymphatics engorged with lymph.

The walls of the lymphatics, in contradistinction to those of veins and arteries, are extraordinarily permeable. Increased pressure within the lymphatics tends to make their walls water-logged. In addition, lymph drains out of the lymphatics into the neighbouring

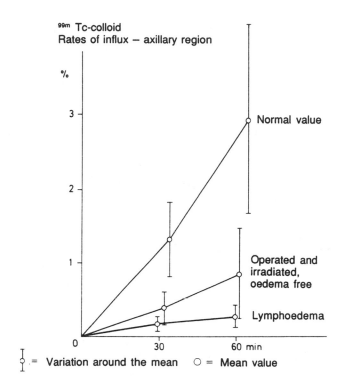

FIGURE 7. After surgery or radiotherapy for breast cancer, transport of radioactive material from the lymphatics is slowed - even when there is no oedema present.

tissues. The stagnant, protein- rich fluid gradually leads to scarring and other changes within the tissues. Hence, after a time, the lymphatic becomes a rigid and inert tube; the lymph congeals in the dilated vessels whose pores are blocked similarly by scar tissue.

It can be readily appreciated that lymphoedema must develop as a result of these changes, since the blood capillaries continue to allow proteins to infiltrate the tissues until the demands on the lymphatics can no longer be met. It is even worse when there is superadded *injury* or *infection*. In the case of injury, arm lymphatics which are still functioning may be damaged; infection can cause lymphangitis after surgery or radiotherapy for breast cancer. No single lymphatic must be put at risk unnecessarily! Injury, haemorrhage, infection all impose a twofold risk - they lead to increased workload as breakdown products from blood and the debris of dead cells and bacteria must all be carried away from the tissues through the lymphatics. Even normal lymphatics can be overtaxed by situations such as these. In addition, reduction in the number of functional lymphatics, that is of the *transport capacity* of the lymphatic system, and the increased workload operate in the same direction and can lead to further retention of proteins in the tissues. This, therefore, is the reason why - with foresight - all patients after surgery or radiotherapy for breast cancer must be warned, in no uncertain terms, about the risks of injury or inflammation.

Thanks to compensatory mechanisms already described in detail, injury and inflammation can easily induce oedema even when it has not yet appeared. Hence we insist that patients after surgery or radiotherapy for breast cancer, even those free of oedema, should adhere to the rules set out in Table 6.

A few additional words about scar tissue in the axilla. As we have seen, this hinders regeneration of the severed lymphatics. Scar tissue is formed when wound infection complicates breast surgery. Irradiation treatment can also lead to scarring - an unavoidable risk if radiotherapy is a necessary part of cancer treatment. (It should be mentioned at this stage that radiotherapy can also have an adverse effect on the nerve plexus lying in the axilla, and which provides the nerve supply to the arm - the so-called brachial plexus - which can lead to further problems). We will deal with this matter in more detail in another section (4.6). Also, rough, jerky and overzealous gymnastic exercise involving the shoulder joint, commenced too soon after operation, can have axillary scar tissue as its consequence.

In the case of lymphatic obstruction, so-called *lymph-venous anastomoses* may develop. Lymphatics grow into the pores of veins whereby the lymphatic obstruction is partly or wholly relieved. This factor certainly plays a part after surgery or radiotherapy for breast cancer. According to one extreme view, lymphoedema of the arm will only arise when, for one reason or another, this compensatory mechanism fails.

However the situation is still further complicated. The damming back of proteins in the tissues to such an extent has disastrous consequences because the body, faced with mechanical failure of the lymphatic system, makes a desperate effort to overcome it. White blood cells, so-called "monocytes" migrate from the blood capillaries and are converted in the tissues to "macrophages" - large scavenger cells. These cells engulf proteins. Every protein molecule which disappears from the tissues in this way lowers the colloid osmotic pressure responsible for oedema formation. Scavenger cells do more. They produce so-called "proteolytic enzymes" which split up the protein molecules into their individual component parts. As we saw in chapter 1, small molecules, the amino acids, which are the building blocks for protein synthesis, do not impose a greater workload as they are water soluble and can be carried away by the blood stream without further ado. Lymphoedema would never occur if this mechanism were so efficient that the whole protein transport burden could be dealt with continuously in such a way. This is *not* the case however. The mechanism is too feeble, and in a way this is valuable. It would be disastrous if the *whole protein load* from the affected region were continually broken down and then rebuilt all over again by the liver.

As a result of these remarks, the readers will be in a position to understand the following by no means simple definition.

"Secondary lymphoedema of the arm occurs after surgery and radiotherapy for breast cancer whenever the normal demands for the transport of protein by the lymph can no longer be met, as a result of reduced transport capacity of the lymphatic system and/or failure of macrophage activity".

The question put earlier: "Why me?" cannot be answered in a single sentence. The number of factors which play a part and interact with each other are too numerous. It could be that patients will hold the surgeon or radiologist responsible for secondary lymphoedema. Their opinion may be that the operation was far too radical, or that the radiotherapy was too intensive. This question has been the subject of much discussion in recent years. Latterly most medical schools have played down a radical approach to breast cancer for cosmetic reasons, largely to avoid the development of secondary lymphoedema, and many have abandoned post-operative radiotherapy. It is not the purpose of this book on *lymphoedema* to go into contentious issues of *cancer treatment*. One of these however is important and we would like to express it very forcibly:

In deciding how extensive radical cancer treatment should be, one point only should be made - cancer treatment should be optimal. In treating cancer, the eradication of the tumour growth must have first preference. The possibility that a swollen arm could be the result, or cosmetic considerations, must not influence oncological treatment.

As will be seen, we are in a better position to treat secondary lymphoedema of the arm successfully. A lymphoedematous arm is incomparably less harmful than a recurrence of cancer! In *Baath's* otherwise outstanding book "Therapeutic Considerations in Treatment of the Female Breast", one can read: "a very swollen arm is rarely seen today because, during the operation, less tissue is removed from the axilla than before, *precisely because of the risk of lymphatic oedema of the arm*". If, in fact, less tissue is removed *"only because of the risk of lymphoedema"*, this attitude is questionable. Each modification of standard oncological treatment requires a twenty year follow-up before a final and definitive evaluation can be made. The surgeon has to prove that a less radical approach does not influence negatively the chances that a *cancer will be cured*. What the lymphologist expects from the surgeon is a good operative technique. In a word, this depends on the surgeon's manual dexterity.

When the arm becomes swollen, do not reproach the surgeon who has performed the operation on the basis of present day medical standards and his knowledge and ability, or hold responsible the radiotherapist who undertook the irradiation treatment. As you have seen, lymphoedema may easily have resulted from a peculiarity of your own body. Any reproach you make is appropriate when, after breast surgery or radiotherapy and before discharge from hospital, someone omitted to inform you of the measures necessary to avoid lymphoedema of the arm.

4.3 What should you do when, after surgery or radiotherapy for breast cancer, your arm becomes swollen? What should you do if your swollen arm suddenly becomes worse?

You must visit the doctor and have a complete medical examination without delay. You must be aware of the fact that not *every* swollen arm will resolve completely. As stated previously, it may point to a local *recurrence* or a so-called axillary metastasis. In this regard you must understand the following - in spite of removal of a breast and the growth within it, together with the axillary nodes, a few cancer cells may be left behind. When the bodily defense is not capable of destroying these cells, they may multiply and obstruct the lymphatics responsible for lymph transport, or exert pressure on those lying adjacent. The recognition of a situation such as this does not pose a problem of any great magnitude for an experienced doctor trained in lymphology and oncology. By inspection and palpation of the tissues he is well fitted to make a judgment. The final decision is made by computerised tomography (CT) or nuclear scanning and, if necessary, by removal of tissue for examination. *If, in your case, it is a question of the so-called "malignant lymphoedema", treatment according to state-of-the-art medical practice must be started without delay and, the problem of the swollen arm takes second place.* Faced with an oedematous arm, doctors are not powerless to deal with the situation. The lymphologist and the oncologist work together. This brings us to an important consideration which we must not overlook. In the presence of lymphoedema, removal of tissue for examination is only absolutely necessary when, by histological$_{(5)}$ examination, it can be determined whether we are dealing with a benign or a malignant process. After removal of tissue from an oedematous arm you will have to contend with an increase in the degree of the swelling, and this risk must be taken only in the most serious cases. Every patient has the right to be informed about the need for invasive medical treatment. When the doctor advises tissue biopsy, it is always appropriate for you to ask why this is necessary. We stress this because it happens, unfortu-

---

(5) Histology is the science concerned with the microscopical examination of tissue; the histologist or anatomical pathologist is in a position to state whether the tissue shows benign or malignant characteristics.

nately, that tissue is removed from oedematous limbs even though it has no bearing on future management. The doctor's answer to the patient's question must be: "Tissue biopsy is necessary to exclude a recurrence of cancer."

It happens sometimes that oedema of the arm secondary to malignancy is the first sign of disease. The explanation is simple - breast cancer causes metastases in axillary lymph nodes and obstructs lymph flow from the arm. This condition can easily be diagnosed by a thorough medical examination. For a "thorough medical examination", the patient must undress completely. The doctor examines the body *(inspection),* and manually *palpates* the area to be examined. If the doctor merely casts a cursory glance at your swollen hand (not even your arm!), and then refers you to the pathology laboratory or X-Ray department, or prescribes treatment, change your doctor!

4.4 The treatment of lymphoedema of the arm

We have said already in the opening section of this chapter that, unfortunately, many women who consult a doctor with a swollen arm following surgery for cancer of the breast are fobbed off. In taking a history from our patients, we note over and over again: "My doctor told me that I have to get used to it, nothing can be done". Sometimes, even more unkindly: "Be happy that you are still alive". This is a great mistake and bad advice, which if followed could have disastrous consequences. Every swollen arm must be treated, and treated early. We have stated already that we reject totally the belief that a difference of arm circumference of up to 5 cm is of no consequence.

We have likened the tissues of a swollen arm to a swamp, and those of a healthy arm to a rippling mountain stream. In contrast to normal tissues which are being continually perfused with healthy tissue fluid, in lymphoedema the various cellular waste products lie stagnating in the tissues. These products, often toxic, impair cell respiration and nutrition and, together with increased tissue pressure, lead to cell damage and fatty deposits. The body further reacts to retention of protein by an increase in connective tissue, and this newly formed material slowly hardens. One can compare these processes to scar formation. Stiffening of the tissues can limit mobility of the arm, even without brachial nerve injury. Spontaneous recovery of chronic lymphoedema of the arm is not possible. On the contrary, we must anticipate deterioration when bouts of infection or cellulitis occur. The hand can swell like a balloon - the arm can reach monstrous proportions, hanging from the trunk like a great log. The result may be total invalidism (fig. 8).

The major reason why adequate treatment for lymphoedema of the arm after breast surgery is mandatory is the regrettable fact that, in a not inconsiderable percentage of sufferers, one is dealing with a fresh occurrence of tumour within the oedematous arm. It is not only a recurrence of the original breast cancer, but a completely unrelated so-called "lymphangiosarcoma" - even more malignant

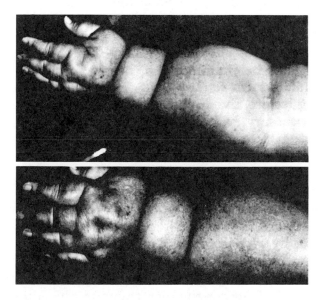

FIGURE 8. Secondary lymphoedema of the arm following surgery and radiotherapy for breast cancer. The fingers are intensely swollen and, on the bloated face of the hand, finger pressure produces deep pitting. There is also doubling of the crease of the wrist. Even at this stage of elephantiasis, it is possible with the the help of Complex Physical Therapy to clear oedema and reach a satisfactory conclusion.

than a carcinoma! If treatment is indeed possible, it is only by removal of the whole limb together with the shoulder girdle ("forequarter amputation").

How should secondary lymphoedema of the arm be treated? In the first place by a thorough examination at the hands of a doctor *experienced in this field.* (Lymphology is only rarely taught in medical schools).

Massage or remedial gymnastics must never be undertaken without full investigation and without drawing up a concise plan of treatment!

We emphasize in this regard that remedial gymnasts are not necessarily trained in either diagnosis or treatment of cancer and lymphoedema. Expert medical consultation begins with a complete case history. Finally the doctor examines the patient - not only the swollen arm but, as we have said already, the whole person, completely undressed. He palpates the operation scar, the axilla, the soft tissues of the shoulder and arm, and compares them with the healthy side; he examines the thoracic organs, the abdomen, etc. *The whole patient is thoroughly examined.* He reads through the referring letters, the discharge summaries and the oncologist's reports. If necessary, he initiates further investigation of blood and skeletal system. In the first instance, his attention is directed to whether he is dealing with a "benign" or a "malignant" lymphoedema, as already discussed. Lymphography and venography are omitted at this stage because these imply diagnostic tests which are not completely harmless, and which may lead even to worsening of the lymphoedema. However there is less controversy about lymphoscintography with isotopes, if expertly performed. If a doctor is confident that he is dealing with a "benign" lymphoedema, he must then decide if initial management should be in a hospital ward, or an outpatient clinic under the direction of a physiotherapist experienced in **Combined Physical Therapy for the Management of Lymphoedema**. Of course other conditions must ultimately be investigated and treated because there are equally important disease states associated with the primary diagnosis, such as cardiac failure, hormonal imbalance and vertebral column lesions which may aggravate the lymphoedema. In this respect the lymphologist treats the patient as would any other specialist.

The kidney specialist or nephrologist, to name one example, has the task of investigating and treating not only the kidneys but also the blood, when there is coexisting anaemia. If it is a question of "malignant" oedema, treatment at the hands of an oncologist is of paramount importance, as already mentioned. Before we deal with Combined Physical Therapy, we will turn our attention to what must *not* be done with lymphoedema. For general measures refer to table 6.

On principle, never allow your swollen arm to be operated on. We classify the indications for operation by defining *absolute* and *relative* indications. "Absolute" implies that only with surgery can the patient's life be saved. It is only justifiable to take risks, including those of anaesthesia, if this is the case. *There is no absolute indication for operative treatment in cases of benign lymphoedema.* One absolute indication is the development of sarcomatous change, but of course we are not dealing here with *benign* lymphoedema.

One speaks of *relative indications for intervention* when, instead of a surgical approach, conservative management is also possible, or when surgery cannot be avoided. After Combined Physical Therapy, in severe cases of lymphoedema the situation often arises when the over-stretched skin of the arm hangs down like an empty sack. One *can* remove this baggy skin, but in no way *must* one do so. This is a relative indication for surgery.

Furthermore the question may arise whether **failed** Combined Physical Therapy should be a relative indication for surgery. The answer to this question is very simple. If the treatment of benign lymphoedema of the arm has been carried out in expert hands, it is *always* successful. It must be emphasized that a large part of Combined Physical Therapy for the Management of Lymphoedema consists of measures which the patient herself must carry out. To be quite precise - if you leave the clinic after Combined Physical Therapy with a recommendation that you wear a suitably fitted compression stocking continually and you neglect to do so, then your arm will swell once again - this is *not* an indication for surgical treatment! No *responsible* surgeon will agree to undertake an operation for lymphoedema on a patient who is unwilling to accept a period of after-care, which may be life-long, and which means amongst other things the need to wear a compression stocking. Or if a patient knowingly works in the garden, incurs injury, and suffers a relapse, this is neither failure of Combined Physical Therapy nor an indication for operation.

If one opts for surgery, the goal should be removal of proliferative connective tissue and fat deposits. In fact, so-called "resection" procedures which aim to remove new formed connective tissue, even at best, leave behind scars. Today some surgeons perform so-called lymph (node) - venous shunts. The surgical attack rests on restoration of the link between obstructed lymphatics and a vein in order to overcome the blocked lymphatic drainage. We have spoken already about such connections occurring spontaneously: nature itself can avert the development of lymphoedema of the arm. Experts often judge the results of these operations very sceptically. Of late even lymphatic transplants have been performed. They lead without doubt to *improvement*, but *one must emphasize here that surgery for lymphoedema is a very specialised field. If, for any reason, you agree to an operation, you should only allow a surgeon highly experienced in this field to operate.* Even the best general surgeons cannot easily perform the occasional lymphoedema operation.

Beware of surgical procedures described by the well known plastic surgeon *Clodius* as belonging to the realm of science fiction! Unfortunately, there are still surgeons who like to treat lymphoedema of the arm with plastic tubes or gauze implants in the oedematous tissues.

If someone recommends an operation called *"venolysis"* give a decisive *no*. In this operation the axillary vein is dissected free from actual or presumed scar tissue. The advocates of this operation do not understand the mechanism which leads to a swollen arm after surgery or radiotherapy for breast cancer. They ascribe this to venous obstruction! They are not aware of the fact that even total occlusion of the vein by thrombosis may not lead to an oedematous arm because dilated collateral veins take over venous flow and, of course, the lymphatic system helps out with its safety valve function. Arm oedema after breast surgery *always* depends on lymphatic obstruction, and obstructed venous drainage, *if actually present,* merely *worsens* the oedema. *Obstruction to lymph flow, not to venous drainage, is the factor to be overcome!* Simple operative freeing of a vein is accompanied by severing of many small veins and lymphatics, and scar tissue soon leads to a return of venous obstruction. In the last analysis "venolysis" is *harmful.* There is no sense therefore in performing venography to demonstrate venous obstruction.

Another quite unrelated situation is seen when severe pain, not relieved by conservative measures, follows injury to nerves of the brachial plexus - a condition which may coexist with the lymphoedematous arm (see chapter 4.7).

Faced with an oedematous arm, you should beware not only of *surgical procedures* but also a variety of *conservative methods of treatment* which are useless, even frankly harmful.

For example, it is particularly mischievous to treat *benign* secondary lymphoedema of the arm with the long term use of *diuretic medication.* Diuretics increase urine output and are one of the most important developments introduced into modern medicine. They are highly effective compounds which, if used correctly, are of fundamental importance in the management of many illnesses. Every medication, along with the desired effect, possesses side-effects. So it is with diuretics. In ordering a drug, a doctor must strike a balance, on the one hand between the goals he wishes to achieve with treatment, and on the other hand possible side-effects. Introduction of a drug must be made in such a way that there is a harmonious balance between its mode of action and the illness to which it is directed.

Diuretics function in the following way: After the tablet has been swallowed, it passes through the mucous membrane lining the digestive tract into the blood stream and thence to the kidneys. It alters kidney function in such a way that more water and salt is excreted than normal. This is the explanation for the opinion, held by most specialists, that diuretics are to be used in those illnesses in which there is a need for salt and water to be removed from the body as a whole. Such a situation exists in so-called right heart failure. The patient becomes oedematous, not only in the legs but often in the subcutaneous tissues of the lower half of the body, and even in internal organs - that is their body retains more sodium and water than normal.

Another example of the sensible use of diuretics for long term treatment is for high blood pressure, in which the doctor must similarly ensure that total body sodium is lowered and, by so doing, blood pressure is reduced. In these serious, life-threatening medical conditions, it is self evident that occasional side-effects of diuretic use must be accepted. Their therapeutic usefulness is disproportionately greater than any damage brought about by occasional side-effects. However in secondary lymphoedema of the arm, the problem is in no way related to a raised body sodium. You are fully aware by now that the decisive factor lies in the fact that the tissues of the arm and the adjacent part of the trunk are clogged with protein material. We do not believe that the swelling can be reduced in size to any appreciable extent by swallowing diuretic tablets. At the point of maximum effect of diuretic therapy, salt and water are excreted so that the net loss of fluid from the blood (of course urine excreted by the kidneys is derived from the circulating blood) leads to a temporary increase in blood concentration, because the other constituents of the blood remain in the circulation. This transient haemoconcentration implies increased protein concentration. You know already from the first chapter that, because of this increase, the force which retains water within the blood capillaries, or draws fluid out of the tissues and into the bloodstream, is increased. There is now competition, on the one hand between proteins held back in the tissues of the arm as a result of lymph stasis, and on the other hand the proteins which circulate in the bloodstream. It is quite easy for oedema fluid within the tissues of the arm to flow back into blood capillaries, making the arm slimmer. This effect must be transient because, through loss of water there is a rise in concentration of proteins stagnating in the arm, and as soon as the diuretic effect has worn off the process goes into reverse. In round two of the contest, the proteins still remaining in the tissues of the arm are declared the winner, and suck back "their" fluid from the blood. The net result - as isotopic studies have shown - is that the removal of material which depends on lymph flow from the oedematous tissues is *delayed* by diuretics, in other words the existing lymph flow is *slowed*. For the swollen arm to retain a reduced girth by recourse to diuretics, they must be taken continuously. In the end, the fate of the arm is influenced in a quite negative way. Tissue concentration of retained proteins, increased artificially, hastens the disease process, one equivalent to widespread chronic inflammation and is responsible for the inexorable progress of the disease. In the truest sense, this is a Pyrrhic victory[6]. According to our experience, patients who regularly take diuretics prescribed for secondary lymphoedema, and continue to do so, feel weak and tired, and happily many - without informing their doctors - cease diuretics on their own account. Contrary to our firmly held opposition to long term diuretic use, we occasionally use this medication as a short term measure, as part of our Combined Physical Therapy.

Many doctors manage patients with secondary lymphoedema of the arm by expressing the oedema mechanically, as sole treatment, while others do so in combination with long term diuretics. Originally, the device made by the firm *Jobst* was employed, but today several others are in use (for example Lymphapress, Lympha-mat).

We will refer to the question of mechanical oedema expressors as one of the options when discussing Combined Physical Therapy. We merely mention the fact here that the area involved in stasis includes not only the arm but the upper outer quadrant of the trunk. It is not our purpose to transfer oedema fluid from one area of stasis - the arm - into another - the trunk. We are totally opposed to treatment with oedema expressors alone, or in combination with diuretic therapy. Rather regretfully, we must make it clear that the

---

(6) *King Pyrrhus of Epirus was victorious in battle over the Romans, but his losses were so great that he did not win the war.*

so-called *"stripping"* or *"wringing"* of the swelling from the arm with the aid of elastic bandages or rubber tubes is still practised. By applying great force, a limb can be manually compressed from below up. The process is very painful, and on this account is sometimes carried out under anaesthesia. In the patients' interests, we must express our opinion at this juncture clearly and unequivocally: *stripping oedema under anaesthesia constitutes professional malpractice!* We also repudiate stripping *without* anaesthesia because this procedure is too rough. In recognition of the well-known fact, described by the Australian lymphologist Casley-Smith, that even light percussion of tissues leads to histologically demonstrable injury to the smallest lymphatics, the swollen arm must not be confused with a bathroom sponge filled with water! Naturally the point of view expressed above when dealing with mechanical expressors is also pertinent here. Stripping procedures for arm oedema belong to the sad chapters of medical textbooks. In 1956 a Dutch phlebologist[7], Van der Molen, described stripping for treatment of the *oedematous leg,* but did not recommend it for the arm. He employed rubber tubes to clear leg oedema only when bandaging had failed, and stressed repeatedly that his technique *must never be carried out under anaesthesia.* Just the same, doctors who strip lymphoedema *from the arm* using rubber tubes cite *Van der Molen* as their authority. From time to time patients report attempts to express oedema from the arm using maximally inflated blood pressure cuffs. This practice is equivalent to "stripping".

When describing Combined Physical Therapy we will discuss the question of compression stockings. The application of stockings is an integral part of *Combined Physical Therapy for the Management of Lymphoedema.* Ordering an arm stocking for persisting lymphoedema of the arm is subject unfortunately to appreciable error. *Secondary lymphoedema of the arm is treated occasionally with heparin injections. We know of no scientific publication which has brought forward clear proof that this form of treatment is successful.* If - *rarely* - the complication of inflammation of a vein (thrombophlebitis) is present, heparin can be used as a temporary meas-

(7) *phlebologist - specialist in veins*

ure. Naturally, cellulitis should not be confused with thrombophlebitis. Cellulitis should be treated with penicillin or a similar antibacterial agent and not with heparin.

A particular form of humbug is so-called *"mesotherapy"* for lymphoedema of the arm. Using a hand-held instrument, constructed specially for "mesotherapy" and resembling a revolver, several cannulas are inserted into the swollen cutaneous tissues at the one session, and through these tubes is injected a "cocktail". This contains a broad spectrum of different substances, the actions of which have not been scientifically proven, either alone or in combination. One thing is certain - these multiple punctures traumatise the tissues, including the lymphatics, and bring about negative consequences (increased lymphatic workload and reduction of whatever transport capacity remains). This has already been mentioned on several occasions.

After discussing in detail what treatment is not appropriate for secondary lymphoedema of the arm, let us now turn to *Combined Physical Therapy for the Management of Lymphoedema*. As its name implies this procedure consists of a variety of physical measures. *The success of treatment depends on a sensible combination of these various physical treatment modalities, any one of which in isolation may not be successful and could even possibly be harmful.* An important component of Combined Physical Therapy is massage. It was first mentioned in 1892 by the well known surgeon *Alexander von Winiwarter* who, even then, referred in his work to earlier authors. Even the so-called "egg of Columbus" derives from Winiwarter. He showed that, in the management of lymphoedema of a limb, the *root of the limb* always takes precedence over its distal portion. It is astonishing, and also sad, that for one hundred years this principle has either been forgotten or studiously ignored. We have mentioned the fact, repeatedly, that water-logging of the skin of the arm by oedema fluid extends also to the upper quadrant of the trunk on the same side, because the regional lymph nodes draining this area lie in the axilla. Not infrequently, the anterior thoracic wall is indurated as a result of deep X-Ray therapy.

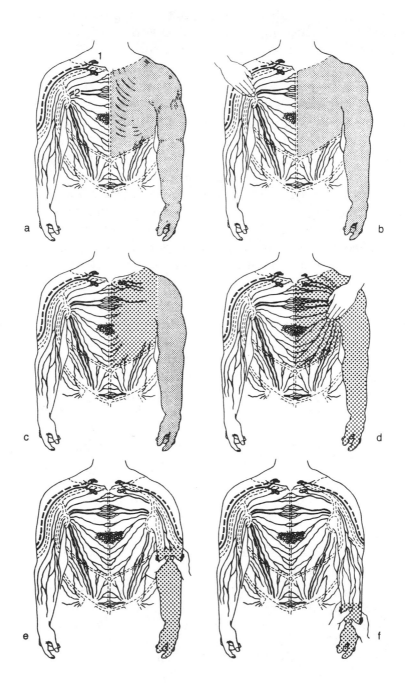

The *first aim of treatment* is directed towards removal of oedema from the upper outer quadrant of the trunk. Over and above its "watershed" function, this region of stasis is connected to the healthy quadrant which lies adjacent to it. Using the *"Manual Lymphatic Drainage"* technique of Dr Vodder, lymphatics are encouraged to accept an increasing workload from beyond their normal drainage area. These draw off oedema fluid, first of all from the area of stasis of the thoracic wall, then finally from the arm and hand further afield (we rightly call these lymphatics "suction vessels"), and carry it away. The scientific basis of this process is the fact that the collecting lymphatics react to a mild mechanical stimulus by increasing the frequency and amplitude of their pulsation **(Figure 9)**. Isotopic venography studies have brought forward proof that clearance of a radioactive substance with affinity for lymphatics and injected into the tissues of the hand of the patient after surgery or radiotherapy for breast cancer is hastened by "manual lymph drainage" from the unaffected quadrant of the trunk.

FIGURE 9.

(a) After surgery or radiography of the left breast, the left arm and shoulder girdle are lymphoedematous. 1) lymph node; 2) lymphatic

(b) The first step in treatment of the adjacent, healthy, right upper quadrant by Vodder's "manual lymph drainage". In this way, the surviving normal lymphatics are stimulated to improve their function.

(c) As a result of treatment described in (b), reduction of lymphoedema has already occurred.

(d) By means of the normal lymphatic drainage, protein-rich oedema fluid is moved carefully from the blocked left shoulder girdle area, across to the adjacent region of the right upper quadrant of the trunk. That means that the lymphatics of the normal side are encouraged to absorb the additional lymph and carry it away.

(e) Rendering the upper arm free of oedema by using manual lymph drainage.

(f) Clearing the forearm using manual lymph drainage (modified after **Kubic**)

In the treatment of lymphoedema, there is a danger that the concept of *"Manual Lymph Drainage"* will become a catchword. *"Manual Lymph Drainage"* is a comparatively recent massage technique developed by the distinguished scientist, Dr Emil Vodder. Used alongside other forms of massage, it has a well-defined place in the management of lymphoedema as part of repeated courses of Combined Physical Therapy. *The implication is that effective management of lymphoedema of the arm is not possible by "Manual Lymph Drainage" alone.* It is very important to stress this fact, otherwise there will be disappointment.

Patients often tell us in their case histories that they were treated unsuccessfully with "manual lymph drainage". Should the patient impart this information to a doctor who lacks up to date knowledge about lymphology, it happens not uncommonly that "manual lymph drainage" is recorded as a worthless procedure and never used again. An additional problem arises when the doctor orders "manual lymph drainage", because he can never be sure that this specialised form of massage will be carried out. Unfortunately it happens repeatedly that, instead of "manual lymph drainage", other varieties of massage are employed - ones which are not only ineffective but can be frankly harmful.

Only after preliminary treatment of the healthy side should further treatment be instigated with the aim of transferring lymph, first from the area of stasis in the affected quadrant, and finally from the arm towards the lymphatics of that quadrant of the trunk previously rendered free of oedema.

It is quite incorrect to try and coax oedema fluid from the arm and into the cutaneous tissues of the shoulder, axilla and chest wall without the prescribed preparation. Such a procedure certainly achieves a reduction in swelling of the arm, but at the expense of increased oedema of the trunk. The net result is chronic inflammation due to artificially induced protein accumulation, which has as its consequence scarring and induration of the tissues. Lymph flow from the arm by way of the superficial skin lymphatics is now obstructed and, through faulty management, the lymphoedema, far from being improved, is worsened. This can be compared with the work of a lazy housemaid who sweeps dust under the carpet.

There are special problems with those patients in whom the cutaneous tissues of the shoulder and chest wall have been indurated by radiotherapy. In these cases the first aim of treatment is naturally to loosen the skin, and this can be achieved to a quite remarkable degree by expert massage. In many cases, after weeks of painstaking scar management, a network of skin lymphatics may appear on the thoracic wall. In this way lymph channels have been opened up once again; this is of great importance for oedema clearance (figure 9).

At this juncture we must deal once again with the place of *mechanical* treatment of lymphoedema. This has an important place in the Combined Physical Therapy as practised by us, but on the other hand we disagree entirely with the *exclusive* use of such devices. The careful reader will understand this attitude. Just as it is inadmissible to undertake the clearance of oedema from the arm without first preparing the trunk, it is both natural and logical to forbid treatment by mechanical means alone. When the shoulder girdle and the trunk are freed from oedema and scar tissue, and when the lymphatics in this region have been prepared, only then can an attempt be made to express oedema fluid manually and then mechanically. The value of treatment with mechanical devices rests solely on the fact that human effort can be spared. In other words, more time is available for the masseur to turn his or her attention to the more important matter of treating the shoulder girdle. The place of apparatus in the Combined Physical Therapy course must be determined individually by the lymphologist and carried out under his or her supervision. Not infrequently, the patient tolerates this form of treatment very poorly and it must be discontinued.

Bandaging forms part of the Combined Physical Therapy alongside manual and mechanical oedema management. Bandaging aims to delay the recurrence of oedema fluid following manual or mechanical treatment, and permits one further component of Combined Physical Therapy, namely *remedial gymnastics*. In every case of lymphoedema there is inevitably a breakdown of those tissues on which normal skin elasticity depends - the so-called elastic fibres. Along with lowering of tissue pressure consequent on effective oedema clearance, this breakdown will result inevitably in reaccumulation of oedema fluid. The bandage raises tissue pressure, and allows remedial exercises to be carried out under strict supervision. These aim to facilitate muscular movement, an important step in oedema clearance. Many patients need to wear their bandages during sleep. If for any reason they leave off their bandages or compression stocking, even temporarily, the arm should be kept elevated. For example, one of our patients has devised a simple suspension apparatus for long car journeys. In the home a bolster can be used. A simple detachable frame can easily be constructed by a carpenter (**Figs. 10, 11**).

Implicit in scientific medicine is the principle that treatment requires *measurement*. In a patient with high blood pressure, the pressure must be recorded at the start of treatment and regularly throughout the follow-up period. In the diabetic, blood sugar and other laboratory tests are basic to good control. In the case of lymphoedema of the arm, the extent of oedema before the beginning of treatment must be measured numerically, and the results of treatment set against these figures. For a day to day check, the arm circumference at pre-determined points is sufficient. For scientific purposes we prefer volume measurement. Even tissue turgor can be measured. In the not infrequent cases where shoulder and elbow movement is restricted, the range of movement can also be measured. Complete return to normal of the condition being treated can only occur during the clearing phase of Combined Physical Therapy if treatment has begun in the first or reversible stage, before either scar tissue or fat has been laid down. If Combined Physical Therapy has been initiated only in the second stage of spontaneous irreversible lymphoedema, stage 1 of oedema clearance must address the problem of removal of the protein-rich fluid which has accumulated. The proliferating connective tissue and adipose tissue remain behind for the time being. To achieve complete return to

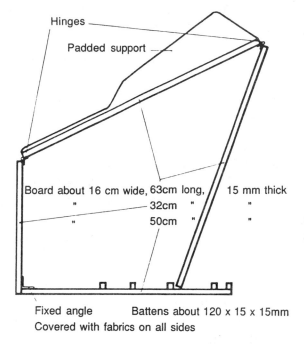

Hinges

Padded support

Board about 16 cm wide, 63cm long,   15 mm thick
          "   32cm   "   "
          "   50cm   "   "

Fixed angle   Battens about 120 x 15 x 15mm
Covered with fabrics on all sides

FIGURE 10. Any good carpenter can devise a simple frame. The affected lymphoe-dematous arm can be rested on this type of support if, for any reason, the arm bandage or compression stocking needes to be removed temporarily.

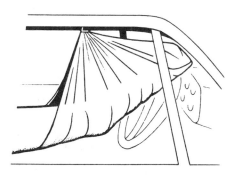

FIGURE 11. For long car journeys, the patient with lymphoedema can find a simply erected arm support useful.

normal requires several years of "phase 2 - Maintaining and Optimising" the results of Combined Physical Therapy.

The duration of the first, that is the clearing, phase of Combined Physical Therapy, whether it has begun in the *first* or *second stage* of lymphoedema, amounts in expert hands to less than four weeks on average. If treatment has commenced in the *third stage of lymphostatic elephantiasis*, the *"first clearing phase"* requires several months. In uncomplicated cases *(stage 1 of lymphoedema)*, Combined Physical Therapy can be carried out in the treatment rooms of a qualified and experienced physiotherapist, provided that daily (even better twice daily) treatment can be guaranteed.

In general, it is useful for a doctor to be able to determine whether treatment options are to be "symptomatic" or "curative". We speak of curative treatment when we are successful in combatting the root cause of an illness. To give an example: the causative organism in lobar pneumonia is the pneumococcus. Definitive treatment of pneumonia requires the administration of a drug which kills pneumococci. Such a drug is penicillin. Before the discovery of penicillin, pneumonia could only be treated "symptomatically". The temperature, usually elevated, was lowered by administrating fever reducing medicines and applying hot poultices. Obviously treatment which attacks the cause is more valuable than treatment which controls symptoms, even though with the earlier symptomatic remedies there is no doubt that many lives were saved.

Does then Combined Physical Therapy for the Management of Lymphoedema attack the cause or relieve the symptoms? **Without doubt, Complex Physical Therapy is the definitive treatment for lymphoedema.** As already explained many times in this handbook, reduction of the normal physiological lymph drainage is responsible for lymphoedema, quite independently of whether it is a question of primary lymphoedema due to a developmental abnormality or secondary lymphoedema. Lowering of the physiological lymph drainage and the transport capacity of the lymphatic system below the normal threshold for protein clearance leads to critical protein stagnation in the tissues. We know from animal experiments that, after injections of homologous blood plasma, a situation develops at the injection site which, in this respect, is analogous to lymphoedema - the picture corresponds to that seen in chronic inflammation. Through *Combined Physical Therapy,* protein stasis is averted and the transport capacity of the lymphatic system is raised to the level of the normal requirements for protein removal.

The same arguments, why bandaging is necessary, explain why, at the *successful conclusion of the first phase of* Combined Physical Therapy, compression stockings are necessary and represent an indispensable part of the second phase of reduction of lymphoedema. It is very hard for many patients to come to grips with an arm compression stocking or a glove because their affliction is now immediately evident to all. There is no escaping the fact that one must compensate for loss of skin elasticity. Wearing a compression stocking need not cause intolerable pressure, or cut off the circulation. After a time most patients find it comfortable. We prescribe made-to-measure stockings and gloves. From our experience, the firm *Varitex* has proven to be the best supplier of compression stockings. Only in exceptional circumstances do we order compression stockings for the arm made out of lighter material. We are often compelled to, however, for frail, elderly people if they are unable to get assistance in applying them. Patients with an injury to the nerve plexus supplying the arm accompanying lymphoedema also tolerate only light weight compression stockings. For patients with paresis of the arm following nerve injury, we prescribe sleeves for the hand and arm, together with splinting and a sling **(Fig. 12).**

This device is indispensible; there is no doubt that oedema may easily recur in the dependent, immobile arm after the completion of Combined Physical Therapy because of failure of the "muscular pump" and the influence of gravity. **Figure 13** shows a simple compression stocking for the arm, with a separate handpiece. With a tendency to more severe oedema of the arm and shoulder girdle, we order arm compression stockings with a top piece and sling **(Figure 14).** For lymphoedema of both arms after bilateral surgical and irradiation treatment for breast cancer, compression stockings with a bolero can be prescribed **(Figure 15).**

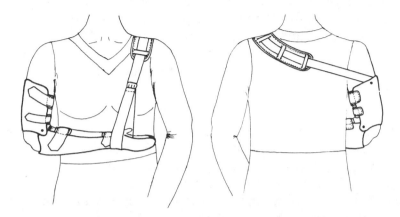

FIGURE 12. Hand and arm appliances for patients with secondary lymphoedema of the arm and brachial plexus palsy. (This illustration, together with Figs. 13-21 and 26-32, were drawn by Frau A. Volmer of the firm Franz Schaub, Freiburg, Germany.)

Figures 16-19 show different types of compression gloves. Figure 20 demonstrates how glove compression can be strengthened. The compression glove with fingers closed at the end illustrated in Figure 21 is made-to-measure by the firm Jobst. We do not use ready-made stockings.

We should not fail to mention that a substantial part of *Combined Physical Therapy for the Management of Lymphoedema* is meticulous skin care for the affected limb, and that the patient must not only learn remedial exercises but must also possess the knowledge required for good skin care and cleanliness. The well known lymphologist Kinmonth has expressed the view that the skin must be kept as clean as that of a surgeon's hands in preparation for surgery. For daily use on the lymphoedematous limb and corresponding shoulder girdle, including for nightly application, we have found one ointment particularly effective - *unguentum lymphaticum (PGM)*. Scars, including those due to radiotherapy, and areas of induration are made more supple with the use of this ointment and painful spasms are quickly relieved.

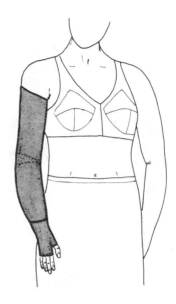

FIGURE 13.
Compression arm stocking
without shoulder extension
but with attached glove

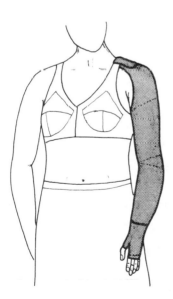
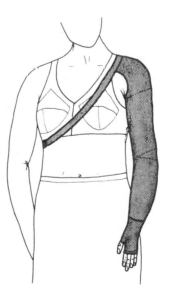

FIGURE 14. (a) & (b): Compression arm stocking with shoulder piece, halter and glove.

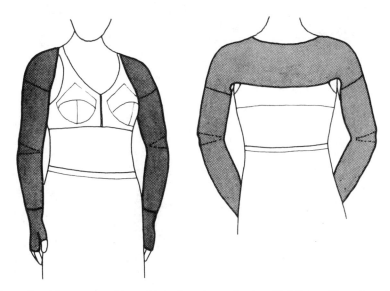

FIGURE 15. Double arm stocking with bolero for patients with bilateral lymphoedema.

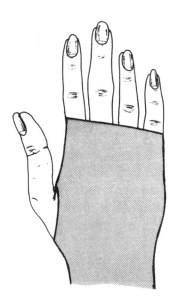

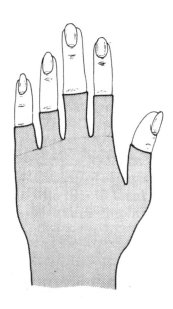

FIGURE 16.
Compression glove without thumbpiece.

FIGURE 17.
Compression glove with short fingers.

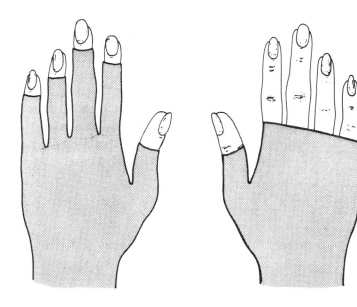

FIGURE 18. Compression glove with long fingers.

FIGURE 19. Compression glove to include the thumb.

These thoughts now lead us to the question of the **second phase** of Combined Physical Therapy which serves to **maintain and maximize** the results of treatment achieved in the first phase. The treatment of lymphoedema of the arm by no means ends with Combined Physical Therapy. To maintain and maximize successful results of treatment, the patient must also make her contribution throughout life. In this respect lymphoedema does not differ from any chronic disease. For those who suffer from obesity, weight reduction achieved in a special weight clinic cannot be maintained if the patient yields once again to the pleasures of cream cakes. Blood pressure will rise again if the necessary medication is not continued and food rich in salt is consumed. We repeatedly remind patients who come to us with lymphoedema of the arm that Combined Physical Therapy makes sense only if, after leaving the clinic, they are prepared to abide by certain rules. Regular manual

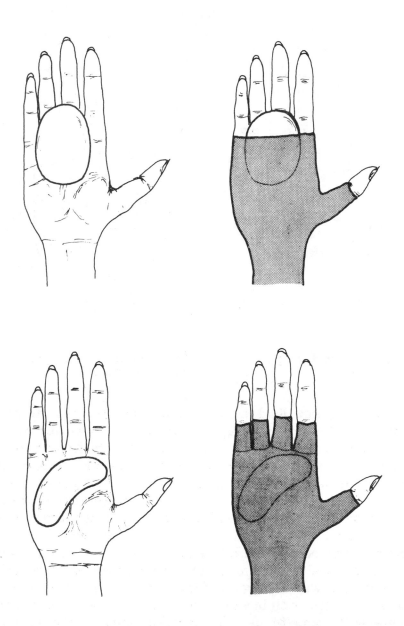

FIGURE 20. "Komprex" compression pads to be worn within the compression glove over the palm and back of the hand.

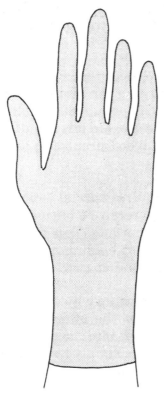

FIGURE 21.
Full finger compression glove

lymph drainage, maybe twice weekly, is always required if the shoulder, axilla and chest wall are to be kept free of oedema. When you have read the descriptions given earlier you will have no difficulty in understanding table 6, as well as appreciating the need to heed the advice given. Your arm can be maintained in an oedema-free state if you follow these rules. Our experience shows this to be true. Furthermore, additional benefit can accrue, in the course of time, through gradual breakdown of fibrous or fatty tissue.

We need not reiterate that injury from a kitchen knife can have serious consequences. The injury leads to loss of blood not only externally, but internally, into the tissues. Inflammation follows, then products of inflammation accumulate and must be carried away by the lymphatics - that is lymphatic workload increases. At the same time, lymphatics which were perhaps still functioning are severed. Infection adds very easily to this situation. Once again lymphatic workload increases and compromises the surviving lymphatics. Lymphangitis further impairs the transport capacity of the lymphatic system.

In taking a history from our patients, we hear repeatedly that after many oedema-free years following surgery for breast cancer, the mere act of carrying a heavy shopping bag or suitcase has led to the sudden appearance of a swollen arm. Here again it is a matter of the disastrous combination of an overtaxed blood circulation and strain on the lymphatic system.

There are two reasons why ironing requires special caution. Ironing is a strenuous task, and one can also receive a burn on the arm. Burns can be regarded in the same way as cuts. This is the reason why we always warn our patients against holding a lighted cigarette in the swollen hand, that is, the hand at risk.

Strangely enough we are often asked by doctors why we are opposed to wearing a wrist watch on the side of the affected arm. The explanation is simple. A watch band can cut into the skin and allow oedema or tissue fluid to ooze out, or it can simply irritate the skin and be a portal of entry for bacteria (**Figure 22**).

It is a wise precaution to wear rubber gloves for household tasks, as they spare the compression glove and the arm stocking and afford extra protection. It is incomprehensible to us as lymphologists that patients after mastectomy are often advised to wear a prosthesis of the same weight as the remaining breast. This unwise advice leads to the supply of a prosthesis weighing one and a half to two kilograms, and the wearing of a brassiere with a shoulder strap which cuts deeply into the skin of the shoulder. Sometimes the band of the brassiere cuts into the chest wall (**Fig. 23-24**). We have already spoken about the cutaneous lymphatic plexus and the anastomotic connections which link the upper quadrants of the chest wall with each other and with the axilla.

We know already what a heavy burden is imposed on the plexus after removal of axillary nodes. The superficial skin lymphatics must remain open at all times to allow drainage of oedema fluid

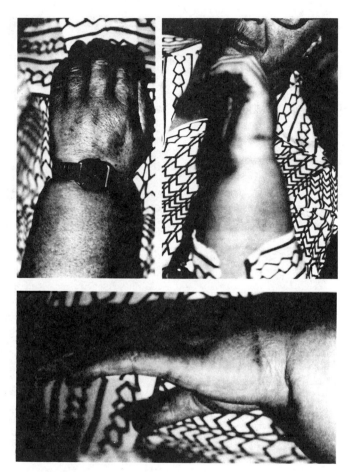

FIGURE 22. The patient with secondary lymphoedema of the arm after surgery and radiotherapy for breast cancer must not wear her wrist watch on the affected arm, otherwise lymph flow from the hand is obstructed and the skin may be injured.

from the arm tissues. A brassiere band which cuts a circular groove in the skin of the chest wall obstructs the lymph nodes which lie between the creases of the groin and the armpit. In health, the area below the navel drains into the groin and that above the navel into the armpit. After removal of axillary lymph nodes the situation arises where the flow of lymph is reversed in the sense that lymph flow from the entire thorax now empties into the lymph nodes of the

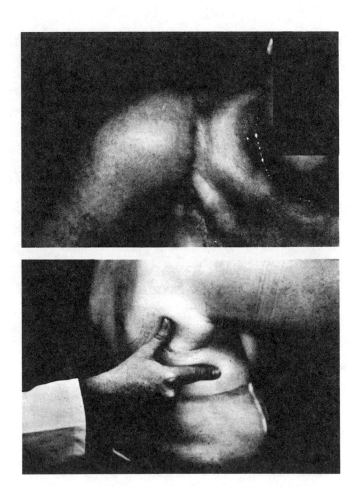

FIGURE 23. A heavy prosthesis and tight brassiere cause further lymphatic obstruction and increase lymphoedema.

groin. We have seen already that, when treating lymphoedema of the arm by manual lymph drainage, the physiotherapist "works" on these lymphatic connections with particular care with the aim of opening up new pathways by artificial means. Clearly it is non-sense to obstruct these lymphatics quite unnecessarily by allowing the patient to wear a heavy prosthesis. In treating such patients,

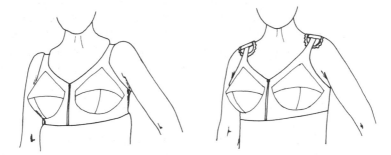

FIGURE 24. Instead of a brassiere strap cutting deeply into the skin (left), lighter cups should be worn. Slipping a pad under the strap gives added protection to the cutaneous lymphatics.

it may save many weeks of effort if we dispense with artificial obstructions to lymph flow such as these. The correct advice should read: "Wear as light a prosthesis as possible, and put padding under the shoulder strap". If you cannot manage a pad of cotton wool, use the *Beiersdorf* model. This is fixed to the thoracic wall and weighs down the prosthesis far less than other prostheses. If the unusually large size of the remaining breast leads to problems, it is wiser to have a breast reduction operation. The best approach is for the surgeon to remove breast tissue and so avert the occurrence of a second cancer.

The reason for the advice given for beauty and body care is self evident. We have spoken already about the need for scrupulous cleanliness as well as basic skin care. Dirty skin is equally important as a risk for the development of bacterial and fungal infection because cellulitis which, even when treated early and successfully, leads inevitably to worsening of the situation. Why the cuticles should not be cut or pushed back when manicuring the nails, and why caution should be exercised when using a nail file, need not be reiterated here because the reason has already been given. Irritating or allergenic cosmetics can lead to inflammation, and you know by now what disastrous consequences inflammation can have for lymphoedema of the arm - by increasing lymphatic workload together with a decrease in the existing transport capacity of the lymphatics. We are also against saunas and sun bathing because, quite naturally, the skin circulation of the affected arm is greatly increased by these activities. Circulation is increased further by exposing even the healthy side to heat, and this leads to yet another increase in lymphatic workload. This does not mean that a patient with a lymphoedematous arm may not enjoy sea bathing on a sunny day. The amount of exposure to the sun's rays when walking from beach to sea is not dangerous. What is forbidden is sun bathing. The patient must use a beach umbrella when lying on the sand. It is not only theoretical considerations which led us to adopt this ban on sun bathing. Clinical experience has taught us that some patients who have stayed out in the sun after surgery or radiotherapy for breast cancer have seen lymphoedema develop within hours, or with other patients have seen it suddenly become worse.

Rough, kneading massage of the swollen arm at risk as well as of the corresponding quadrant of the trunk, which is usual in sports massage, is to be avoided at all costs. *Winiwarter* has already warned us about masseurs who "proudly display bruise marks". A bruise is caused by torn blood vessels through which blood flows into the skin and, when blood vessels tear, the more delicate lymphatics are damaged to a considerably greater extent and in far greater number. To repeat a technical dictum used by lymphologists, *"rough massage raises the lymphatic workload and reduces the transport capacity of the lymphatic system"*.

A patient who, after surgery or radiotherapy for breast cancer visits the hairdresser, whether lymphoedema is present or not, should protect herself against direct heat both before the drying process and when under the hood. This requires no further mention. In many patients ignorance on this subject was the very reason for lymphoedema developing, or why the lymphoedematous arm became worse.

The reason we ask for special care in the garden is obvious. Neglect of this advice is very often the factor which precipitates lymphoedema. Unfortunately women who take pleasure in gardening are hard to convince that a simple prick from a rose thorn can have disastrous consequences.

Those who are not cat lovers will find it difficult to understand how a patient who is deeply attached to her cat, and who is advised by her lymphologist to give it away, is reluctant to do so. The advice once given by us to have the cat "de-clawed" surgically can no longer be espoused by us as the Society for the Protection of Cruelty to Animals[8] has threatened us with legal action. Cat scratches can be the cause of quite dangerous infections or inflammatory conditions, and can thereby bring on lymphoedema or worsen it.

The points made in relation to sport need not be reiterated. Quiet swimming is particularly useful. The deep, rhythmical respiratory movement of the thorax brings about a decidedly therapeutic effect. Tennis playing (and also golf) is harmful on account of the strenuous, and often sudden, backward movement of the arm during the "back swing". Nordic skiing is recommended rather than the considerably more risky downhill skiing.

Of considerable importance is the fact that obesity is one risk factor leading to deterioration of lymphoedema. Every kilogram of surplus body fat requires additional lymph flow. Fat laid down in the arm mechanically hinders lymph flow in the delicate lymphatics and slows the production of lymph entering these vessels. For this reason a weight reduction regime and maintenance of ideal body weight is important for the overweight. A high fat diet appears to be harmful to patients who have undergone breast cancer surgery. One recommendation is to restrict fat intake to not more than 25% of available calories. **There is no specific diet which is beneficial for lymphoedema.** A simple, well-balanced diet, rich in vitamins and with restricted salt, is the only dietary advice which one should follow. It is nonsense to suggest that pork is harmful. Many recommend protein restriction - as though it were possible to reduce by this means the protein held back by sluggish lymph flow in the affected arm. The so-called *"Mayr diet"* is nonsense. If one were to reduce the serum proteins by dieting, it would increase (!) lymphoedema. Fortunately, serum proteins do not decrease as a result of the usual dietary measures. In this respect it should not be overlooked that, based on our present knowledge, no diet exists

(8) *Bund gegen den Missbrauch der Tiere e.V.*

which is guaranteed to prevent a recurrence of cancer - or its secondary spread. Unfortunately, alternative medicine and the lay press espouse many and varied "cancer diets". In lymphoedema of the arm, nutrients should be low in salt, because salt leads to water retention in the body.

It is quite harmless to enjoy tea or coffee, and the avoidance of alcohol is not recommended. The quantity of fluid consumed should be governed only by thirst, and not be any prescription. Unfortunately, quite erroneous advice is often given that fluid should be restricted. Smoking should be avoided by every patient.

We have discussed already the need for arm stockings, physical exercises under supervision and compression bandages for night-time use.

A single insect bite can result in such serious inflammation in the tissues involving the lymphatics that it can initiate, or aggravate, lymphoedema. It is commonsense therefore for regions which are insect prone such as Lappland, Greenland and the tropics to be avoided.

In Table 6 we have mentioned a rather delicate subject. It has been stated many times already that the medical profession possesses only a fragmentary knowledge of lymphology. For the reasons given, affected patients have to be informed about which medical procedure and investigation may lead to worsening of lymphoedema. *Should a doctor wish to undertake such procedures the patient must decline!* Blood pressure should not be measured on the affected, that is the swollen, arm. Blood and lymphatic capillaries must not be put at risk needlessly. In the case of bilateral mastectomy with lymphoedema, blood pressure should be measured in the thigh. Of greater importance however is the avoidance of injections, whether hypodermic, intramuscular or intravenous, into the arm or shoulder girdle at risk and already oedematous, and injections into the elbow or shoulder joint are forbidden. It is easy to understand why such injections can damage the tissues or harm the lymphatics and thereby aggravate lymphoedema. Intravenous injections and infusions are particularly hazardous, because lymphatics are embedded in the walls of the veins and may easily be injured by needle puncture. A few drops of fluid may inadvertently be injected outside the vein - "extravenously": at the same time there is an escape of blood into the tissues (more work for the lymphatics); the lymphatics lying adjacent to the veins are damaged; inevitably, oedema worsens as a result of phlebitis (inflammation of veins) or periphlebitis (inflammation surrounding the veins). **Notwithstanding the manufacturer's directions**, "Iskador" should not be injected either into the operation scar or in the axilla. These regions and their lymphatic vessels should be protected at all costs. We need not reiterate that blood should never be taken from a vein, or by finger prick, on the affected or swollen arm, nor should acupuncture or any type of procedure be permitted if it involves puncturing the skin of the swollen arm or shoulder girdle at risk. A problem may arise when, after bilateral mastectomy for cancer, both arms are oedematous and a blood specimen is required or a drug needs to be injected intravenously. In such cases an attempt must first be made to find a suitable vein in the foot. Only when this fails, and a blood specimen must be obtained, should one ignore this injunction.

The final recommendation in table 6 is to seek medical treatment at once should a red inflammatory area appear on the affected arm and be accompanied by fever and chills - an early sign of cellulitis. Please be especially careful to bring these matters to the doctor's attention. Unfortunately we have found that, in the time frame of a brief consultation, the arm is not examined, only the "clinical triangle" sounded, the spot diagnosis of "flu" made, and aspirin or some similar drug prescribed (figure 25).

4.5 - Lymphangiosarcoma or angiosarcoma (Stewart-Treves syndrome)

The appearance of *painless reddish spots resembling small haemorrhages* on an oedematous arm should immediately arouse the suspicion of sarcomatous change. Lymphangiosarcoma or angiosarcoma affects only those patients with grossly neglected and untreated lymphoedema. The best prophylaxis against this life

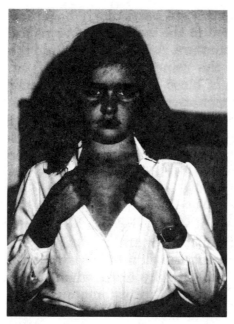

FIGURE 25. The "Clinical Triangle". If ausculation is carried out on a febrile patient only in this area, the diagnosis of cellulitis can easily be overlooked.

threatening complication is correct management of secondary lymphoedema of the arm, that is expertly performed Combined Physical Therapy. If you find a suspicious area or mark on your arm, go at once to a doctor *trained in lymphology*. He will then arrange for removal of tissue for examination. If histological examination confirms the diagnosis, amputation must be performed. This is the only possible way that life can be saved. Lymphangiosarcoma (lymphosarcoma) metastasizes early. Unfortunately, lymphangiosarcoma (lymphosarcoma), because of its comparative rarity, is understandably not known to all doctors.

4.6 Nerve injuries after surgery and radiotherapy for breast cancer

The network of nerves supplying the arm *(the brachial plexus)* lies in the armpit in close relationship to blood vessels, lymphatics and lymph nodes. In the case of severe lymphoedema, the vessel wall and the tissues which envelop the nerves of the plexus are easily involved in the water-logged condition which we call oedema and, later, in the indurated newly formed connective tissue. Symptoms and signs of involvement of the brachial plexus - "brachial neuropathy" - only occur however in a fraction of cases in which radiotherapy is combined with surgical clearance of the axilla. It is due principally to involvement of the blood supply of the individual nerves.

A brachial plexus lesion can lead to disordered sensation, pain, muscular weakness, even paralysis (even the most severe oedema never causes paralysis *on its own*, that is without irradiation injury, and never unbearable pain). We should add that, apart from this *benign* mechanism, the cause of the lesion can be metastases from breast cancer. In summary, the doctor's first task is to make a sound diagnosis.

Brachial plexus injury accompanying lymphoedema adds to the difficulties of treatment and compression bandaging. The lesion itself is notoriously hard to manage. For this reason, such patients must be treated in a clinic in which all relevant specialist services are at the disposal of the treating lymphologist. In circumstances where there is severe pain, the operative treatment recommended by *Clodius* should be used in order to give the patient freedom from pain, particularly if there are also motor deficits, as progression towards paralysis can then at least be halted.

In rare instances a carpal tunnel syndrome may accompany lymphoedema, and in these cases X-ray treatment is rarely the cause - more commonly it is lymph stasis - in other words the oedema itself. The small carpal (wrist) bones and the anterior ligament form a tunnel. The median nerve passes through this tunnel into the palm and, because of oedema, can be subject to compression. Characteristically, the carpal tunnel syndrome is associated with pain in the hand (occasionally radiating to the shoulder) and paraesthesia. Expert Combined Physical Therapy can be very successful, and surgery is often avoided.

4.7 Irradiation damage to the skin

Ulceration can occur in the anterior chest wall and axilla as a result of severe irradiation injury. This is in no way amenable to conservative treatment and should be left in the hands of a good plastic surgeon. Unfortunately, alternative medicine practitioners may try useless procedures, like ozone injections, which achieve nothing except a waste of valuable time. Coexisting lymphoedema will not be aggravated to any extent by surgical treatment, however postoperative manual lymph drainage is a requisite. The considerably less serious condition called *irradiation telangiectasis* (dilatation of small blood vessels) also requires plastic surgery because, if left alone, skin cancer may develop.

4.8 Secondary reconstruction of the breast

This term implies breast reconstruction *following* radical mastectomy for cancer. (In primary breast reconstruction, a plastic surgeon is part of the surgical team carrying out radical mastectomy. The breast is reconstructed *immediately* so that the patient waking up from anaesthesia does not have to suffer the severe psychic trauma of loss of a breast). This technique should only be practised by a careful, experienced surgeon. The lymphoedema is not expected to be any worse after this type of operation, just the same it is recommended that a course of manual lymph drainage treatment be instituted following the reconstruction procedure, and this also facilitates wound healing.

4.9 Disability pensions

A woman who suffers from secondary lymphoedema of the arm after surgery or radiotherapy for breast cancer may still be severely disabled, even when her arm is rendered free of oedema by successful treatment in the clinic. She must strive, daily, to maintain this oedema free state, observing a whole list of "do's and don'ts" which have an impact on her lifestyle. Information about the requirements for certification for a disability pension can be obtained from the appropriate social security office in your state or country.

5. SECONDARY LYMPHOEDEMA OF THE LOWER LIMBS AND EXTERNAL GENITALIA FOLLOWING SURGERY AND RADIOTHERAPY FOR MALIGNANT DISEASE

Should you have to undergo treatment for malignant disease, for example cancer of the uterus or prostate, lymphogranuloma (Hodgkin's disease) or removal of lymph nodes, or should you receive radiotherapy in this region, the lymph drainage from the lower limbs, the lower abdominal wall up to the navel, and the external genitalia may be involved. In the case of a malignant tumour (eg. melanoma, sarcoma), the lymph nodes of the groin must also be removed. Why this is necessary is known already to the reader from previous discussion. After clearance of lymph nodes from the groin, there is obstruction to lymphatic drainage from the leg and the lower abdominal wall on the operated side up to the umbilicus.

The attentive reader who has digested the chapter on secondary lymphoedema of the arm after surgery or radiotherapy for breast cancer can answer the question why lymphoedema can occur after treatment of cancer of the lower abdomen, and why many patients are spared this condition.

After removal of lymph nodes, the transport capacity of the lymphatic system is reduced drastically, however a total and absolute block never occurs. Yet, even when all connecting lymphatics are removed, the intrinsic skin lymphatics, the cutaneous prelymphatic channels and those in the walls of the blood vessels may still remain open and guarantee a link with adjacent draining areas of the trunk. The lymphatic system is still intact. In exactly the same way as after clearance of axillary lymph nodes, the body strives to overcome any serious interruption of lymph flow by processes of restoration (collateral circulation, anastomoses between lymphatics, new connections between lymphatics and veins) and naturally, in these cases, the macrophages play their part. Only when these mechanisms fail will lymphoedema develop.

Lymphoedema can also appear immediately after surgery or radio-therapy and, by virtue of the restorative processes mentioned earlier, can ultimately recover. Lymphoedema may also recur after a latent interval, which may be months or years. In other cases, cancer treatment is not followed by lymphoedema but, after an oedema-free interval of perhaps many years, it once again manifests itself. Once again the explanation is fatigue and insufficiency of overworked and worn out collateral vessels, coupled with failure of macrophage activity. Of course an additional disease process which leads either to an increased lymphatic workload or reduced transport capacity of the lymphatic system (or, as usually occurs, both together) suddenly tips the balance and upsets the fragile equilibrium which allows lymphoedema suddenly to appear. We have seen that even an insect bite may be sufficient provocation.

In spite of the fundamental similarities between the problems of lymphoedema of the upper and lower limb after surgery or radio-therapy for cancer, there is a difference which we would not like to pass over without comment. We have seen that venous obstruction is rarely a factor in the development of a "swollen arm" after clearance of axillary lymph nodes. On the other hand, leg vein or pelvic vein thromboses are dreaded complications of abdominal and pelvic operations. For this reason, it is very likely that a swollen leg in the early post-operative period points to venous obstruction and not to lymphoedema. (We will see in chapter 6 that inadequacy of the lymphatic system does play a very definite part in the development of oedema due primarily to venous thrombosis). In the overwhelming majority of cases, deep vein thrombosis occurs during the period of hospitalization. This usually poses no problems to the doctor; leg or pelvic vein thrombosis, unlike lymphoedema, is no stranger to the surgeon and appropriate treatment will soon be instituted. Nevertheless there will be errors from time to time, and post-operative lymphoedema may be misdiagnosed as deep vein thrombosis and treated with a prolonged course of anticoagulant therapy. This potentially dangerous treatment is not indicated in lymphoedema. The concept is widely held that, after the so-called Wertheim radical hysterectomy for uterine cancer, followed by radiotherapy, a swollen leg is seen only when leg vein thrombosis is the underlying factor - that is "pure" lymph stasis can never be held responsible for the swelling of the leg. This attitude is false. One should urge the greatest restraint in ordering venography or lymphography for a leg vein thrombosis ("DVT") after surgery or radiotherapy for malignant disease in this region. If such a course is recommended, the patient should make sure that the precise indication for this investigation is made quite clear. If the oncologist or gynaecologist regards the investigation as indicated *for assessment of the cancer itself*, then the patient must be made aware that the procedure carries a risk and that the swelling could become much worse. Moreover, when secondary lymphoedema occurs after cancer treatment, the underlying factor may be a recurrence of the tumour. In the treatment of deep venous thrombosis the results of venography or lymphography may make no difference to management, and therefore it is unacceptable to take a potential risk knowing that the swelling may increase. We have no objection to isotopic lymphography, that is when technetium is used as the radioactive marker. Isotopic lymphography with radio active gold is no longer used as it may also lead to an increase in the swelling.

In contradistinction to primary lymphoedema of the leg, which in the great majority of cases begins distally in the foot and ankle and spreads from there to the groin or lower abdomen, secondary lymphoedema after surgery or radiotherapy for cancer of the organs mentioned above commences mainly in the upper part of the thigh, sometimes the external genitalia as well, and then gradually extends down the leg. Once again, we must state emphatically that lymphoedema of the lower limb, for anatomical reasons, very often involves the lower abdomen. It has far reaching consequences for treatment, and is unfortunately poorly understood by many doctors involved with the treatment of diseases of the lower extremities.

The reader who has noted carefully the chapter on secondary lymphoedema of the arm after surgery and radiotherapy for breast cancer will understand clearly that, in the first place, a sensible approach to lymphoedema of the leg is careful decongestion of the lower abdomen and groin by manual lymph drainage. A quite inexplicable misunderstanding about this basic principle leads to the application of unphysiological, and often harmful, procedures.

We refer to the "stripping" with elastic tubes referred to on page 72. This compression technique starts at the metatarsal heads at the base of the toes and proceeds proximally. A prominent vascular surgeon spoke about this compression technique (which has its own number in the medical benefits schedule) as follows: "The oedema fluid displaced is so obvious that, at the upper end of the compression bandage, a massive collar of oedema can be recognized". This "spare tyre" of oedema, involving the root of the limb and the tissues of the lower part of the trunk, results in bursting of the severely overtaxed lymphatics; lymphoedema already present in this region is increased or, if not already present, it now appears for the first time. Lymph stasis and protein build-up will bring about a vicious cycle of chronic inflammation, new connective tissue formation and fibrosis, as you know already. Quite often, in patients treated with this stripping technique, we can identify a band as hard as gristle across the root of the limb which effectively blocks lymph drainage from below. The physiotherapist may frequently have to struggle for weeks to loosen up this region manually and, unfortunately, does not always succeed in restoring to normal the condition which existed prior to treatment. The same remarks apply equally well to the various mechanical means of oedema clearance. With regard to progression through the various clinical phases of lymphoedema, there is no difference between leg or arm oedema, or between primary and secondary lymphoedema.

Surgery and radiotherapy may be followed, at first, by a latent interval in which there is no oedema. After months, perhaps years, *reversible* lymphoedema may develop. This progresses through a *spontanenous irreversible stage,* and finally to the stage of *lymphostatic elephantiasis.* The risk of sarcomatous degeneration is also present. Bouts of inflammation (cellulitis) are also a frequent accompaniment of lymphoedema of the leg.

We ask the reader interested in details of management to read through section 4.3 on secondary lymphoedema of the arm after surgery or radiotherapy for breast cancer. The management of the oedematous leg is identical in this respect; the treatment of choice is *Combined Physical Therapy for the Management of Lymphoedema.* After thorough hygenic measures, those lymphatics lying in the lower quadrant of the trunk adjacent to the area of stasis are encouraged, by cautious manual massage, to accept a greater workload. The second step is to transfer oedema fluid, little by little, from the oedematous lower quadrant across to the normal side. Finally the limb is cleared of oedema - first the thigh, then the leg and finally the foot. Bandaging, gymnastic exercises and elevation of the limb also belong to the realm of Combined Physical Therapy.

The treatment of lymphoedema of the genitalia poses a particularly difficult problem. When the tissues overlying the pubic region are indurated by radiotherapy, often with deep, transversely running contractures, one must concentrate initially on freeing them. This is often extraordinarily successful - the cutaneous tissues once again become supple and pliable. In our clinic we are accustomed to apply *ung. lymphaticum* for this purpose. It is often necessary to start with definitive oedema clearance by more intensive manual lymph drainage before the actual genitalia are treated. Naturally, the second phase of maintaining and optimizing the successful results of Combined Physical Therapy follows closely on the first. The made-to-measure compression aids must be ordered. **Figures 26-32** show the various stockings and compression hosiery, occa-

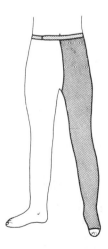

FIGURE 26. Compression stocking with one-sided support.

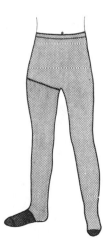

FIGURE 27. Combination type pressure hose.

sionally of the combination type. Exactly as for lymphoedema of the arm, it is only possible to achieve normality by phase 1 of Combined Physical Therapy when treatment has begun in the first stage. If connective tissue proliferation is already present, a return to normal cannot be expected solely by phase 1 treatment, but will occur during phase 2 of *maintaining and maximizing improvement*.

In Table 7, the reader will find guidelines which must be followed if those suffering from lymphoedema of the leg wish to maintain optimum improvement. It is self evident for every reader who has understood the foregoing discussion that injury must be avoided at all times, or at least as far as possible. Every injury has a double impact on the condition - the lymphatic workload increases and, at the same time, the transport capacity of the lymphatic system is proportionately reduced.

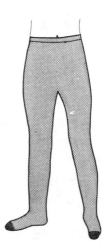

FIGURE 28. Compression hose
with a double stocking and foot pieces.

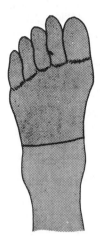

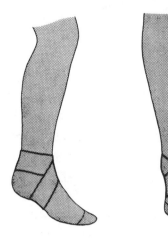

FIGURE 29. Elastic sock
with individual toe pieces.

FIGURE 30.
Criss-cross bandaging.

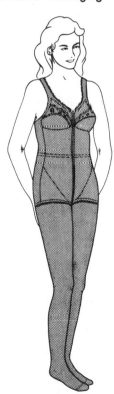

FIGURE 31. Compression hose
and elastic corset.

TABLE 7. Recommendations for patients with lymphoedema of the leg, or when it is threatened.

1. Avoid injuries.

1.1	Do not wear tight or high-heeled shoes or constricting buckles. If you have been ordered orthopaedic fitted and padded shoes, wear these only.
1.2	Never walk outside barefoot (risk of injury).
1.3	Take care with podiatry. Do not cut the cuticles.
1.4	Use no irritating or allergenic cosmetics.
1.5	Never permit injections to be given into the skin, muscles or joints of the affected leg.
1.6	No acupuncture! No leeches!
1.7	Avoid regions prone to insects when on holidays.
1.8	No frostbite! (Wear socks in cold weather).

2. In the case of fungal infections of the toes (cracks between the toes, yellow brittle nails),visit the doctor without delay!

3. In the case of bacterial infection or infectious illness, visit the doctor immediately!

4. If you notice a bluish red discolouration of the skin, or haemorragic spots on the affected skin, visit the doctor immediately!

5. Carry out remedial gymnastic exercises regularly, wearing your compression stockings or pantyhose. Always wear the compression hosiery ordered by the doctor.

6. No saunas!

7. No sunbathing!

8. Floor heating is not recommended in your home.

9. Never overstrain. Quiet swimming is theraputic.

10. Your nutrition:

10.1 Maintain a desireable weight.

10.2 Have a well-balanced diet. (Meat, vegetables, fresh fruit)

10.3 Reduce salt intake.

11. For dressing:

Briefs with bands which cut into the skin, or which leave behind creases, should not be worn. Combination pantyhose are preferred. Do not wear tight belts!

12. During sleep, keep the oedematous leg elevated or bandaged.

13. For women - consult your lymphologist concerning family planning.

14. For those with flat feet or splayed toes - wear orthopaedic insoles.

15. Do not sit with your legs crossed.

16. Kneading type massage of the lymphoedematous , or potentially lymphodematous, leg is not allowed.

17. Do not allow a vascular surgeon to inject or remove varicose veins!

Regarding footwear (1.1), high-heeled shoes greatly restrict upward and downward movement at the ankle joint, thereby reducing, for practical purposes, the pumping action of the calf muscles and movement of the ankle joint itself. Both reduce venous blood flow and increase lymphatic workload. Narrow "court" shoes with pump soles effectively cut into the skin and obstruct lymph flow, thereby worsening the already existing tendency for the toes to become oedematous and consequently for fibrous tissue to be laid down (Fig 33). One should never walk outside barefooted (1.2) because this would invite injury, and this injunction holds particularly for the seaside.

The pharmaceutical company, Janssen, gives the following advice for those who suffer repeated fungal infections:

1) Use clothing and footwear which minimize sweating.

2) Wear only underclothes which can be boiled.

3) Change daily, particularly if you have been perspiring.

4) Avoid walking barefoot in critical areas, such as indoor swimming baths and change rooms.

5) Do not leave bath towels on "infected" floor areas; if you do, use a fresh towel to dry yourself.

6) Start drying yourself from the head down, the feet last.

7) Use foot baths where provided.

8) Avoid alkaline soaps.

9) Maintain general bodily hygiene.

10) If these instructions are not successful, use an anti-fungal cream preferably on feet and toes, taking care always to dry between the toes. Treat with antimycotic preparations, or dust your socks with powder, or both.

Any appearance of reddening of the skin accompanied by fever and chills is suspicious of cellulitis, and you must visit the doctor

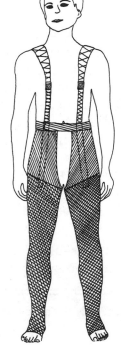

FIGURE 32. Wrinkle-free double compression hosiery with hip fastening for men or women, with inbuilt braces made from rigid material. This specially handmade "Varitex" stocking with hip support was devised by the authors in collaboration with members of the orthopaedic factory of Franz Schaub, Freiberg. Illustration - A. Vollmer, Freiberg.

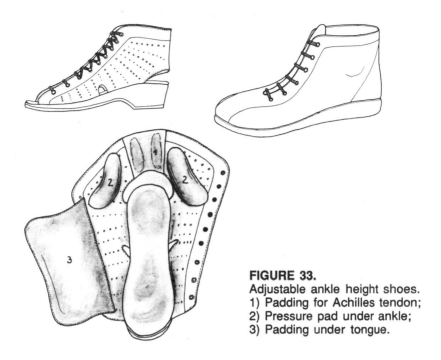

FIGURE 33.
Adjustable ankle height shoes.
1) Padding for Achilles tendon;
2) Pressure pad under ankle;
3) Padding under tongue.

without delay so that appropriate treatment can be started. If you are leaving on holiday, ask your doctor to prescribe suitable medication to take along with you.

Remedial exercises form part of the maintenance and aftercare measures required after treatment in the clinic for clearance of oedema. Always use the prescribed compression devices. If your lymphologist has ordered bandages for night-time use, make sure that you use them.

Saunas, sunbathing and floor heating increase lymphatic workload (6,7,8). Rough, kneading type "sports massage" is harmful as it causes an increase in blood circulation with consequent increase in lymphatic workload. Bruise marks left behind by the masseur implies injury to blood capillaries. Blood which oozes into the skin represents increased lymphatic workload, and of course lymphatics as well as capillaries are injured (16). All strenuous exertion is

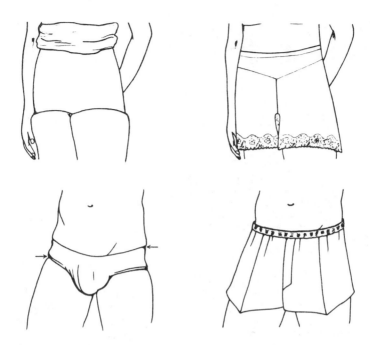

FIGURE 34. Briefs showing incorrectly constricting (left) and correct (right) waistband.

harmful. Swimming, as long as it is not competitive, is good therapy for lymphoedema.

As already mentioned, there is no specific "lymphoedema diet", and the principle should be - maintain your weight; obesity aggravates lymphoedema. Take a normal, well-balanced diet and keep your salt intake low (10). It is not sensible to be thirsty!

Take careful note of point number 11, that is appropriate clothing. Neither men nor women should wear briefs or any underwear which have an elastic waistband. A visible groove should never be seen after removal of underwear as this blocks lymphatic drainage. Tight belts are also harmful - you must be free to breathe. Do not wear socks which leave creases under the free edge. Do not wear tight jeans which constrict the waist or the body (Fig 34, 35).

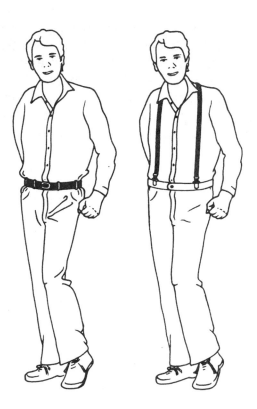

FIGURE 35. Narrow belts (left) are harmful as they obstruct lymph flow and constrict breathing.
Right: comfortable trousers and braces.

Pregnancy is risky for the patient with lymphoedema of the leg; consult an expert lymphologist if you are planning a pregnancy (13). Orthopaedic abnormalities aggravate lymphoedema. If you are ordered insoles, wear them (14). Never sit with crossed legs - this interferes with venous flow and leads in turn to increased lymphatic workload.

Above all, when the limb is already oedematous or a recurrence is threatened, it is our recommendation that after you have mastered phase 1 of Combined Physical Therapy and have entered the second phase, you should attempt to build on and maintain what you have achieved in phase 1 and commence ambulant manual lymph drainage together with remedial exercises. Occupations which require that you sit or stand for prolonged periods are not suitable for patients with lymphoedema of the legs, and we recommend a change of occupation or retraining. In view of the frequency of occlusive arterial disease of the legs, it is often found to coexist with lymphoedema. On no account permit endarterectomy or any other arterial surgery. This will only allow lymphoedema to worsen - lymphatics always fall victim to vascular surgery. Claudication pain will automatically improve with the compression treatment necessary for the lymphoedema (table 7, point 17).

6. THE OEDEMA OF CHRONIC VENOUS INSUFFICIENCY OF THE LEGS

It is not the aim of this book to give a detailed description of venous insufficiency of the legs, yet, considering the frequency of this complaint, we must give our readers some guidance on the subject. We are limiting ourselves however to those conditions which form an inseparable part of lymphology, and with which patients suffering from lymphoedema should be conversant.

"Chronic venous insufficiency" is not a diagnosis but a description of a pathological condition to which several diseases of veins can contribute. It can include development abnormalities, a severe varicose condition, or the aftermath of a deep venous thrombosis ("DVT") - *"post thrombotic oedema"*.

In chronic venous insufficiency there may be a serious disturbance of venous haemodynamics$_{(1)}$ of the affected leg *during walking*, but there is normal blood flow at rest. The expert speaks of *"ambulatory venous hypertension" and "hypervolaemia"*$_{(2)}$. Pressure in the leg veins is raised considerably during ambulation and, as a consequence, much blood is retained in the veins.

The reader who has read carefully the opening chapter of this book knows that an increase in venous pressure must lead to increased pressure in the blood capillaries. As a consequence, filtration pressure is raised so that an increased quantity of fluid leaves the capillaries by ultra-filtration and appears in the interstitial tissues as an *increased lymphatic waterload*. The noble lymphatics leap eagerly into the breach with their safety valve function and *compensate*, for the time being, for this onslaught. However the moment that the lymphatic waterload exceeds the transport capacity of the still healthy lymphatic system, a state of (as yet) *low protein oedema* arises as a consequence of this *dynamic failure*. We name this special form of dynamic failure *"dynamic veno-lymphatic"*, and

(1) haemodynamics: the study of the basis of blood circulation

(2) hypervolaemia: increased circulating blood volume

it leads to a situation where the causative factor of *this type* of dynamic insufficiency is disease of the veins.

The clinical picture of this oedema due to venous-lymphatic-dynamic decompensation is characteristic. The sufferer gets up in the morning with a slim leg which steadily swells during the course of daily *ambulant* activity. When he or she retires for the night, pitting can be produced by finger pressure over the ankle and shin. During the night the oedema disappears. Remember that there is no disturbance of venous haemodynamics in the recumbent position, only when walking.

The only rational treatment for this condition is by *compression* - either by bandaging the leg or the use of a *highly efficient compression stocking (not just support stockings)* ordered by the doctor. Compression must be maintained at all times when on your feet, but can be removed when you lie down.

The sufferer who has steadfastly worn his or her compression stocking throughout the day, takes it off at night and can see with satisfaction that the leg has *not* swollen. The onset of oedema has been forestalled. Manual lymph drainage *is not indicated* in this condition, but just the same it is not contra-indicated. It is not forbidden, rather it is unnecessary.

We must stress at this point that *medical treatment is no substitute* for compression therapy, and indeed so-called "thrombosis" medication, alleged to*"protect against oedema"* or to *"strengthen capillaries"*, or the use of *diuretics,* are not valid alternatives. Between these two groups there is a fundamental difference. The "oedema preventing" medications are in fact *harmless* (many help to control oedema) and can be used as adjuvant therapy, that is in conjunction with compression, as well as for long term use. For example, when for any reason occlusive arterial disease accompanies chronic venous insufficiency and compression is not possible, there is no other course except to use these "vein" preparations as sole treatment on a long term basis. It is, however, utter nonsense to treat chronic venous insufficiency with *diuretics* - a form of stupidity which the purveyors of these preparations with a turnover of several millions have introduced and promoted by extensive advertising. To treat oedema limited to one leg with a substance whose action is targeted on the *kidneys,* and which is capable of severe *side effects*, is comparable to shooting a sparrow with a blunderbuss. (We hope that the animal welfare agencies do not threaten us with legal action over this remark). To do this not once, but day in, day out for years and even decades is crazy.

Advertising by one of the drug companies depicts a woman's slim and shapely leg - wearing a high-heeled shoe! She is accompanied by a young charmer in evening dress wearing a brightly colored top hat (he represents the firm's diuretic tablets). The leg is "tapped" in the manner of a beer keg. Oedema fluid gushes freely from the leg. Indications for this treatment are among others "problems of stasis" (!) in the legs as a consequence of fluid collection (oedema) arising from venous obstruction. A particular advantage is specified, in that the diuretic tablets work throughout the day, so that at night both the treatment and the patient can be rested. With his index finger raised, the charmer declares why this is so. "It is nature's will".

Side effects (the law requires that side effects must be listed) are really trivial:

> "As a result of disturbances of water and electrolyte metabolism, hypovolaemia and circulatory disorders such as headache, giddiness, visual symptoms, circulatory weakness, confusion and disorders of coagulation as well as, in rare cases, cramping pain in the calf ... deteriorating metabolism in the diabetic can require modification of diet or dosage of antidiabetic medication. In certain patients there may be a rise in uric acid leading to the clinical picture of gout. Potassium deficiency, particularly where dietary potassium is low, vomiting or chronic diarrhoea ... hypocalcaemia ... rise in blood lipids ... a rise in urea or creatinine; disturbances of hearing; pancreatitis ... loss of appetite ... digestive disturbances (nausea, vomiting) ... in exceptional cases there may be changes in the red blood corpuscles (megaloblastosis). Allergic reactions (exanthemata), rarely anaphylactic shock; changes in the blood

picture (anaemia, leucopenia, agranulocytosis, thrombocy-topaenia) ... various reactions in certain individuals may affect their ability to drive a vehicle or be in charge of machinery. This occurs for the large part at the beginning of, or change in, medication as well as when alcohol is consumed."

The whole charade costs (when ordered in bulk) merely 63.5 Pf$_{(3)}$.

We would like to clarify another point for our readers - *varicose oedema cannot be eliminated either by injecting or operating on varicose veins, and in the presence of oedema these measures are contra-indicated.* If you wish to have your varicose veins treated by blocking injections or by operation, make sure that you are informed of the possible side-effects and risks, and note that cramps in the calves are not caused by varicose veins$_{(4)}$.

In the treatment of *leg cramps,* therefore, neither injecting nor removing varicose veins should be considered. In most cases, a compression stocking can be worn instead of injection or surgical treatment.

A recent judgment of 14/11/87 (AZ:VIZR 65/87) of the German Federal Court is a salutory lesson. The issue at law was whether conservative management of a knee cartilage condition diagnosed as chondromalacia of the patella should have been offered as a reasonable alternative to surgery:

"If there exist several comparable medically indicated and commonly practised methods of treatment which have indentifiable risks and chances of success, it is thereby understood that, for the patient, a choice is possible, and the patient must be permitted, by means of appropriate and detailed explanation on the part of the doctor, to make a decision regarding which way treatment should be directed and what risks are entailed in this treatment".

(3)   *currently around $US 0.45*

(4)   *Translator's note: Dr Földi points out that the German word for varicose veins - Krampfader - does not mean "cramp" but is based on an Old High German word meaning crooked - "crooked veins".*

In this case there is an abundance of treatment options which should be tried before surgery, namely *medical treatment, physiotherapy,* or the ordering of *special shoes* with low heels.

In principle, identical problems are presented by a degenerative condition of knee cartilege and by varicose veins. Complications can arise even after an injection in the buttock, albeit rarely. The medical journal "Medical Tribune" recently called upon all doctors to take note of the law and explain to patients even why injections need to be administered. One thing is certain - there is no danger with compression treatment!

Once again, we must reiterate that in the presence of lymphoedema or lipoedema, injections or surgical treatment for veins is contraindicated. On the one hand the condition can deteriorate, on the other hand compression treatment required for lymphoedema or lipoedema can help the veins at the same time.

If compression treatment is not carried out the condition will continue to deteriorate still further, even though the limb has been kept dry artificially by the misuse of diuretics. Lymphatics as well as blood capillaries overloaded by ambulatory venous hypertension are injured, so that initially purpuric spots, and later a brown pigmentation of the skin, will involve the calf region. The oedema becomes *protein enriched* and no longer resolves with bed rest. A gradual and progressive connective tissue proliferation leads to a horny induration of the skin and the subcutaneous adipose tissues *(lipodermatosclerosis).*

Our well-informed readers know already that it is no longer a matter of *safety valve function.* To emphasise that veins are the cause, we are pleased to use the term *"phlebolymphatic insufficiency".* Often a leg ulcer will develop - *"varicose ulcer of the leg".*

This late stage of chronic venous insufficiency is an indication for Combined Physical Therapy. Carried out expertly and with the patient's cooperation, even "spat" ulcers will heal. If, however, footdrop has developed as a late complication, this must be treated surgically.

7. LIPOEDEMA AND "CELLULITE"

Lipoedema is a characteristic clinical condition seen in women, unrelated to lymphoedema, and of unknown cause. Even though the upper part of the body remains slim, both legs are severely affected by symmetrical fat deposition so that they resemble riding breeches, the swelling extending from the pelvic girdle as far as the ankle. There is often a hemispherical, fatty pad in the inner side of both thighs at knee level. The dorsum of the foot is spared.

The affected parts are often tender to pressure but, in addition, firm pressure with the fingertip will lead to bruising - in other words bleeding into the skin. During the day, towards evening, oedema develops over the instep and lower calf; finger pressure now causes pitting. The oedema clears with a night's rest.

The arms as well as the legs may show this same symmetrical lipoedematous condition.

There are many interesting analogies between lipoedema and the so-called "cellulite". The characteristic manifestations of the latter condition ("peau d'orange"[1], mattressing, etc.) occur almost without exception in lymphoedema. "Cellulite" is regarded by many authorities such as Professors *Ryan* and *Curri* as not a trivial complaint, not even as a *neologistic disease*, nor as *"prematurely aged female skin"*, but as a genuine illness which, instead of the lay term *"cellulite"*, should be termed *"panniculitis oedematosclerotica"*. (We ask our readers who wish to question their doctors about the subject to refer them to the book written by T.J. Ryan and S.P. Curri, "Cutaneous Adipose Tissue", published in 1989 by Lippincott Press, Philadelphia, USA). It is not by chance that cosmeticians have treated *"cellulite"* by manual lymph drainage for decades with a degree of success.

---

(1) *"peau d'orange" (orange peel) has been the traditional term used in medicine for the appearance of the skin in this condition, due to cutaneous oedema.*

There are several reasons why we have included a discussion on lipoedema in this book:

1. It is always confused with lymphoedema.

    The most important difference between lipoedema and lymphoedema, as far as the patient is concerned, is that the lipoedema may reach the dimensions of elephantiasis and restrict mobility drastically, thereby interfering with the patient's livelihood, but it never becomes malignant.

2. Lipoedema is often incorrectly managed.

    Occasionally weight reduction is advised, but this is of no value. Lipoedema is a disease of abnormal adipose tissue ("Kummerspeck"[2]) whereby the body metabolism diverts calories into fat. (There are actually cases in which lipoedema and obesity coexist - it can be a cause of adiposis dolorosa; in these cases a reduction diet is necessary to remove surplus fat.)

3. Another error is prescribing diuretics for this condition.

    These certainly prevent oedema formation, but have no effect on lipoedema and lead, after prolonged misuse, to severe side effects.

4. Surgical removal of adipose tissue is a major procedure which carries a not inconsiderable risk. By damaging lymphatics it can lead to lymphoedema. We warn our readers against *lipectomy*.

5. So-called *"liposuction"* - a rather brutal method of "curetting" adipose tissue after breaking it down with the aid of a jet pump - must be condemned. Several fatalities have been recorded already.

(2) *Translator's note: Kummerspeck - lit. "pained blubber" has no colloquial English equivalent. In medicine it is termed "adiposis dolorosa".*

6. There are many important correlations between lipoedema and lymphoedema. The fact that lipoedema may be associated with orthostatic$_{(3)}$ oedema implies that the lymphatics in the lipoedematous leg become inadequate for the task by the latter half of the day. An adequate lymphatic system precludes oedema. With increasing years, many cases of lipoedema change to a mixed form - "lipolymphoedema". It would be beyond the scope of this book for us to get too involved with this extraordinarily interesting topic.

With the patient's co-operation, *Combined Physical Therapy* may be effective in lipoedema, just as in lymphoedema. By the same token, an intensive phase 1 treatment of about 4 weeks duration is required, leading directly to the second phase of maintaining and maximizing the earlier good results. In lipoedema a compression stocking must invariably be worn. It is often astonishing how the adipose deposits melt away under compression and the leg once again becomes shapely.

Lipoedema can be found in conjunction with a variety of other diseases. As mentioned already, there is a combination of lipoedema and obesity.

Lipoedema can also be associated with orthopaedic conditions, for example osteoarthritis of the knee. It is sometimes found in association with venous insufficiency of the leg. There are patients in whom multiple combinations are seen, e.g. lipoedema plus lymphoedema, chronic venous insufficiency, osteoarthritis and obesity. In expert hands extraordinary success may be achieved even in cases of this nature and, in the majority, encouraging early results can be maintained and even improved.

We hasten to warn patients who suffer from lipoedema against sclerosing injections or surgery for varicose veins. Those who suffer from lipoedema are very much at risk of developing lymphoedema. It would be a great pity if varicose vein operations carried out for purely cosmetic reasons were to be followed by lymphoedema.

(3) orthostatic: resulting from the upright posture

APPENDIX 1

1. Movement therapy for reduction of oedema in patients with lymphoedema of the upper and lower limbs

Oliver Gültig and Hans Pritschow

Introduction

Movement therapy and exercises for the reduction of oedema form part of Combined Physical Therapy and are necessary to maintain the successful results of this treatment. Muscle activity (contraction and relaxation) as well as joint movement (hips, arms and spinal column) exert a profound influence on the lymphatic system.

Guidelines for your movement therapy

In order to prevent injury, when carrying out therapeutic exercises you should adhere to a few guidelines, as follows:

1. Individual exercises should not induce pain, not even discomfort.
2. Jerking, lurching or straining is not allowed.
3. Exercises should not be too stressful, nor should they lead to any muscle stiffness.
4. Every active phase (maximum 5 seconds) should be followed by a break of equal duration (5 seconds).
5. During arm or leg movements, the arm or leg respectively should be kept elevated.

A few tips

Do not carry out your exercises in bed (it is too soft). Take a blanket and lie on the floor.

Begin with a few exercises only, and then gradually increase the range.

Do your exercises daily, even twice daily whenever possible.

The total time for which you exercise should not exceed 20 minutes.

Exercises carried out with bandaging in place will intensify lymphatic activity because your muscles are working against the resistance of the bandage.

A few suggestions and possibilities for movement therapy.

a) <u>Exercises for loosening up and relaxation.</u>

As a starting point for the proposed arm or leg exercises, you should begin every session with exercises for relaxation and loosening up.

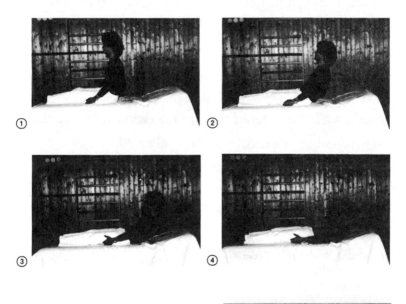

In a sitting position, let your head hang forward loosely. When the tension in your back muscles loosens, go down slowly and lie on your back.

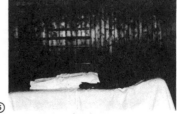

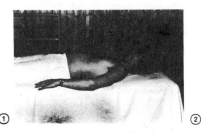
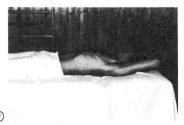

Breathe in and out using your abdominal muscles. When breathing out press your lumbar spine against the blanket.

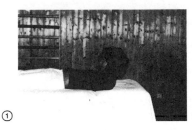
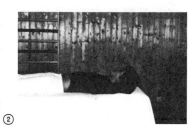

Breathe out with more force, raise your head, then lay it back again.

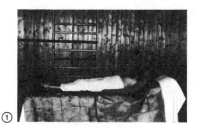

Breathe out, press your lumbar spine against the blanket. Breathe in and relax.

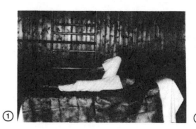
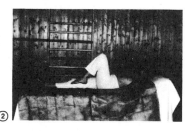

Breathe out forcibly, flex your knee, breathe in, put your foot down again, first the right and then the left.

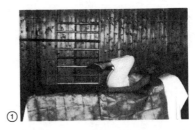

Breathe out, flex both knees. Breathe in and straighten your legs again.

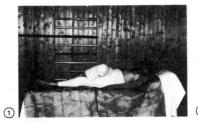 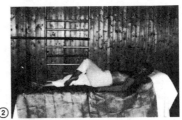

Flex your right knee and move it across the thigh. At the same time twist your head to the right. Relax, then repeat for the other side.

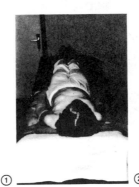 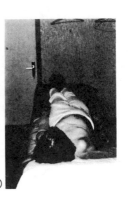

Final position lying straight on your back.

Breathe out, slide your left hand towards your left knee. Breathe in and return to the original

b) Exercises for the lymphoedematous arm

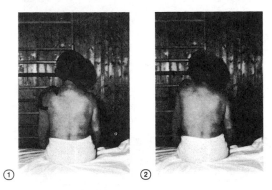

(1) Shoulder circling.

(2) Raising and lowering the shoulder

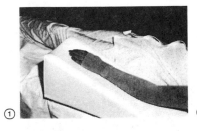 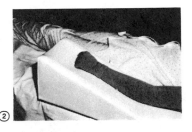

(1) Starting position

(2) Firmly close and open your fist

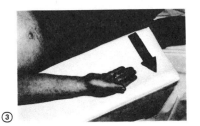

(3)

Lay the back of your hand flat on the floor then return to starting position.

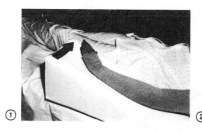 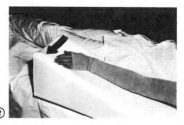

Move your hand towards the thumb side and then towards the side of the little finger.

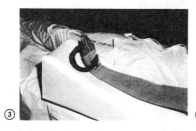 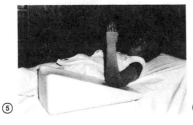

Hand circling

Breathe out, press your whole arm against the wedge support. Breathe in and relax.

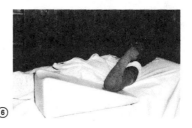

Raise your forearm and lower it again.

Move your forearm up and down towards your shoulder.

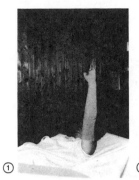

① Raise your arm vertically and lower it again. (Careful, do not allow your arm to fall to your side).

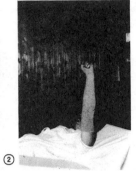

② Arm vertical, make a fist and open it again.

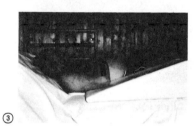

③ Breathe out, press your arm against your chest. Breathe in and relax.

c)   Exercises for the lymphoedematous leg (with compression bandage)

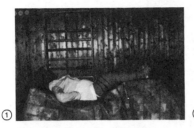

① Starting position

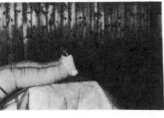

② Stretch your feet, press your calf against the wedge support

③ Raise your foot and bend your toes towards you

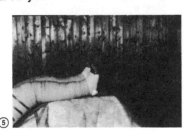

④ Claw your toes

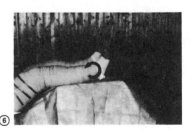

⑤ Spread your toes wide

⑥ Foot circling, in and out

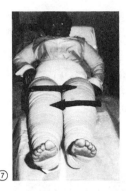

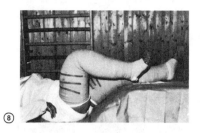

Breathe out, press your knees together. Breathe in and relax.

Raise your right knee then straighten it.

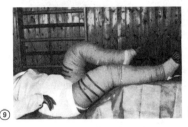

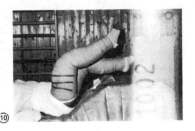

Raise your left knee then straighten it

"Riding a bicycle"

129

d) <u>Movement therapy in water (water temperature 31-34 deg.C)</u>

The buoyancy effect of water means that your joints are not weight bearing, they move more easily (they float). The hydro-static pressure means that movement is against resistence and the warmth of the water relaxes the musculature.

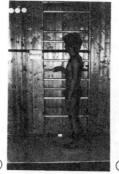
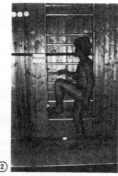
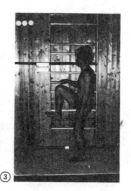

Starting position.

Raise the left knee and stretch it.

Raise the right knee and stretch it.

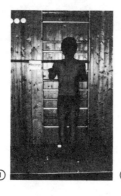
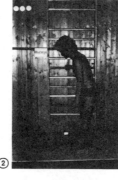
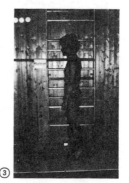

Stand on tip toe with both hands on the horizontal bar. Return to starting position.

Stand on your heels.

On your toes and back again.

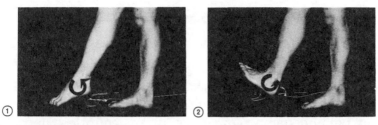

Foot circling in and out

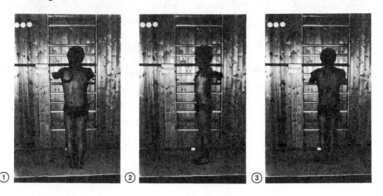

Both hands on the bar, relax one hand, raise the arm to the horizontal and back again to the bar.

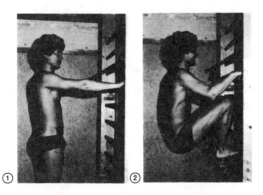

Both hands on the bar, bend your knees and stretch again.

CONCLUSION

We do not claim that the proposed set of exercises is complete. It is more important to show you that what you do can have a positive effect on your lymphoedema. Your body affords countless opportunities for varying these exercises. Take these hints and suggestions as a guideline and "create" your own individual movement therapy to achieve reduction of oedema.

If you are at all uncertain whether you should or should not carry out a particular exercise, your masseur or remedial gymnast can help you.